It's *Not*
Carpal Tunnel Syndrome!
RSI Theory and Therapy
for Computer Professionals

First Edition
Printed in the United States of America
Published by Simax, Philadelphia, PA
February, 2000

Library of Congress Catalog Card Number: 00-90189
ISBN 0-9655109-9-9

Foreword

The sharp upswing of soft tissue disorders among workers in the electronic workplace has caught us all off guard. From regulatory agencies and the insurance industry, to health professionals and the patients we treat, huge numbers of people are struggling to comprehend and combat the problem. The trend is all the more surprising because it is occurring in work that appears to be less physical, whereas nerve, muscle, and tendon problems of the upper extremity have historically been associated with work that is overtly physical. In their aptly titled, *It's Not Carpal Tunnel Syndrome*, Suparna Damany and Jack Bellis apply principles of physical therapy and ergonomics to resolve this seeming discrepancy.

Damany, an experienced physical therapist, and her co-author, Bellis, a long-time computer-user and recovering patient, focus on non-surgical treatment and prevention of RSI. They do so through an informed overview of RSI's many diagnoses, the content of common therapies, and the rationale behind physical medicine interventions. It's Not Carpal Tunnel Syndrome is not a tome of patho-anatomy or physiology, and the authors wisely avoid the controversies that surround RSI and other soft tissue diagnoses, such as fibromyalgia. Rather, their point of origin is that structured dynamic therapy—putting the body in motion and making it fit for keyboard work—along with posture and keyboard techniques, often resolve clinical syndromes that have traditionally been the domain of orthopedic surgery. As such, they are proponents of a new and evolving model that is as important in today's medical repertoire as non-surgical management of low back disease was a generation ago. For instance, a number of key concepts, pointed to by Damany and Bellis, are upheld by practitioners who treat office-related soft tissue injuries. These include 1) the importance of posture in causing musculo-skeletal disorders; 2) the preference of dynamic treatment over splints and medication; 3) the prevalence of nerve compression in the chest [thoracic outlet syndrome, or more specifically, "transient proximal nerve compression"] for many upper extremity symptoms; and 4) the need for a continuum of techniques in the treatment regimen, from mobilization to strengthening. Not long ago, these concepts and measures would have been assigned to the dustbin of alternative therapies. Now, there is growing acceptance of their value.

It's Not Carpal Tunnel Syndrome is composed in the model of a resource guide, with excellent sections on the use of the Internet, informative books and articles, and preventive and therapeutic exercises. For those with symptoms, it can be used as a primer on what to expect from therapy, and perhaps even more important, how to assess therapies that may be incomplete or inappropriate. Whether you are a new or chronic patient, a therapist, or a manager interested in prevention, It's Not Carpal Tunnel Syndrome will serve you well.

Martin Cherniack, M.D., M.P.H.
Director, Ergonomics Technology Center of Connecticut
Professor of Medicine
University Of Connecticut School of Medicine

Preface by Suparna Damany

I've been a physical therapist for twelve years. Over that time I've treated patients for injuries both related and unrelated to work. In recent years, my work has focused on repetitive strain injuries because of what has become an avalanche of cases. Sadly, many of these cases involve misunderstood symptoms, misdiagnosed conditions, and worse yet, misapplied surgery. Because RSI is only starting to be accurately understood, it's likely that many of these unfortunate patient experiences may have been inevitable.

But the evidence is mounting to present a clear picture that explains computer-related RSI, and my experience with many patients has made it clear to me that the problem involves chronic muscle and nerve involvement of the entire upper body. For long-term computer users, any other view is likely to be shortsighted. It's time for the medical community to incorporate this information into its collective pool of knowledge. This book is my contribution toward that goal.

When I started treating RSI, my patients' average age was in the mid to upper thirties. Recently however, I've seen the average age dropping, with an increase in the number of RSI sufferers in their late 20's. This is probably because people have started using computers earlier in school and at work, and for a greater proportion of the time. So it's becoming increasingly urgent that we start a mass education program about RSI, reaching into our schools and vocational institutes. This has to start with a change in attitude, move forward with better information, and continue indefinitely with new ways of working. Prevention is a difficult sell, but it is ultimately the most important message we have. If our ideas find their best audience in current RSI sufferers, we call on these individuals to spread the word and help those around them understand the larger logic of RSI that we have presented.

Suparna Damany
Master of Science Physical Therapy (MSPT)
Certified Hand Therapist (CHT), Hand Therapy Certification Commission
Certified Ergonomic Assessment Specialist (CEAS)

Preface by Jack Bellis

I am an RSI sufferer... or is it *victim*? After years of full-time computer work, including various programming jobs and technical writing, I started having problems with my forearms and fingers. First it was aching, then burning, then pins-and-needles, and finally numbness. I postponed dealing with it until I was forced to; my department was about to be disbanded, so I had to get the workers' compensation claim opened while I still had a job. I was referred to an orthopedic surgeon who specialized in hand problems. To make a long story short, I eventually had surgery on one of the nerves in my arm, near the elbow. The day after the surgery, it seemed like I was unconditionally cured—that's how dramatic the improvement was. I felt I had a new "lease on life." But after a few months of typing again, my symptoms returned, exactly the same as they were before!

A year passed before Suparna Damany was brought in to our 400-person software company to institute an RSI prevention program and provide hands-on therapy to employees who needed it. In five minutes of one-on-one consultation, she opened my eyes to RSI phenomena of which even my hand specialist surgeon was apparently unaware. (Or, if he was aware, he chose not to investigate these conditions in my various examinations.) Suparna showed me that I had muscles in a constant, unnatural state of tension, and fibrous knots of tissue accumulated on the nerves that go to my fingers. After several months of therapy to solve these problems and improve my work habits behind the keyboard, I am now in control of my RSI instead of vice versa.

Having read several books on RSI, I was amazed that none seemed to present the same picture that I got from Suparna, to explain how it all fits together. Certainly, many of the books address the same issues and touch on some of the same therapeutic techniques that Suparna employs, but none put the pieces together to address computer-related RSI as a distinct phenomenon. I felt that I must share the message that has helped several of my co-workers, and this book is that message.

In the course of writing this book, the information itself started to take on its own life, coalescing into a general theory of how RSI affects hard-core computer users. Like physicists searching for the elusive "unifying force," Suparna and I have glued together a general scenario that brings together into one explanation the myriad of syndromes and symptoms that comprise RSI. Our message, laid out over the remainder of the book is as follows:
1) Your RSI can be healed, or in the most difficult cases, at least made

manageable. 2) Most of the syndromes that are regarded by traditional diagnosis as the cause of your problems, such as the infamous carpal tunnel syndrome, are actually symptoms not causes. Consequently, you must revitalize your entire upper extremity to fight off RSI. 3) A certain "profile" predisposes some individuals to more serious RSI, including an obsessive work style, perfectionism, and a high number of years behind the keyboard. Identifying these telltale signs of high susceptibility to RSI in certain individuals is important, so that they are not allowed to cross the line from moderate trauma to chronic damage, which takes much longer to heal.

Acknowledging at the outset that we will present many of our ideas in the framework of this unifying theory, we want to state that we will try not to fall into the trap of "monolithic thinking." This is the phenomenon where an author seems to explain everything under the sun in the context of his or her dissertation. Although we will generalize about RSI-prone people, we know that not all computer users are the same, and that many RSI mysteries are still unsolved. So we will try to readily acknowledge where our information blurs, and where you must continue the fact-finding on your own.

We'll just leave you with one more thought, a brief note from a Web traveler, who came across our theory on our web page, www.RSIProgram.com:

> "I very much appreciate your web site. I have been suffering for years, but in my shoulder, not elbow or hands. Your site provides valuable information, much better than most others which only scratch the surface of RSI."
>
> -- Web Visitor

Comments like this make us optimistic that many answers to the RSI puzzle are contained in the following pages, and we hope you find your own answers here, as well.

One may go wrong in many directions,
but right only in one.

—Aristotle

Acknowledgements

Thank you, Susan, Jessica, Kira, Kartik, Akshay, Krish, Alice,
Ann Marie, Tracy, Ellen, Tammy, Charles, Kathryn, Greg, Nita,
Poser, and Copernic for your participation and support.
Without you, this book would not be possible.

Contents

Medical Disclaimer: See A Licensed Medical Practitioner

This book is an educational publication. It is not a substitute for medical advice or treatment by a licensed practitioner and should not be used as such. It is intended only to provide information that will help you interpret and evaluate the information you get from your doctors. *If you have health problems, consult a licensed medical practitioner immediately.*

Every effort has been made to ensure that the information in this book is accurate, but many of the concepts discussed in this book concern conditions that are still very much the subject of debate and speculation. The authors, editors, and publishers disclaim any and all liability or responsibility for damages, consequential or inconsequential, direct or indirect, arising from use of the content of this book. The authors make no warranty, expressed or implied for the accuracy or usefulness of the information in this book, and are not responsible for omissions, errors, inconsistencies with other sources, or misrepresentations.

Part 1: Introduction

RSI and Our Goals

Repetitive strain injury and *cumulative trauma disorder* are terms still being defined, not by the medical profession, but by the community of patients suffering from their effects. Both terms refer to injuries that are caused by the passage of time combined with both physiological and environmental causes. Depending on whom you talk to, RSI can sound like a form of fraud perpetrated by malcontent, malingering employees bent on abusing the Workers' Compensation system, or a debilitating complex of nerve and muscle disorders caused by repetitive work done with the hands. To us, and to anyone who has experienced RSI's pain, numbness, and loss of strength, it is quite emphatically the latter.

Whether one term is better, or will in fact prevail is immaterial. Is it *repetitive* or *cumulative*? Is the trauma always *stress*? Is it an *injury* or a *disorder*? We will spell out a scenario that might best be called *cumulative and constant tension complex*, but the name is of little significance in evaluating the situation and of even less consequence to sufferers. For our purposes, it is all of these things, but we'll use "RSI." After all, our goal is not a better acronym but a successful therapeutic strategy. Furthermore, we will focus on how RSI attacks hard-core computer users. This book is about computer-related RSI.

> We asked one of our case study patients, "Did your doctor's measures help?"
>
> "In the long run, yes. Specifically, because he granted me a prescription to obtain physical therapy from Suparna."
>
> -- Patient B.

Who is this Book for?

New Patients   This book is directed, first and foremost, at those who are most likely to benefit from it… long-time computer users who have just noticed some aches or pains. These individuals are at a critical crossroad and must choose which direction to go. Should they regard their problem as a minor, isolated incident or a sign of something more troubling? What specific actions should they take? We will provide the information to make the right decision and take the appropriate action.

Chronic Sufferers   An equally important audience is comprised of individuals who already know that they have a serious RSI problem, but have been unable to solve their problem. Although they've followed the "conventional wisdom" of improving their ergonomics, working in the neutral position, and taking breaks, this has not been strong enough medicine for them. We believe that what they read here will provide the critical missing pieces of the treatment puzzle.

Prevention   We will also describe prevention techniques to make your individual workstation or entire workplace safer from the ravages of RSI. This information is the most important type of information we can provide because it has the potential to stop the suffering before it even begins. This portion of the book will be of interest to every computer user and people responsible for running offices where computers are used as the primary means of performing a job. As we begin a new millenium, it's clear that this includes a rapidly increasing proportion of workers.

Therapists   Lastly, we hope that all healthcare professionals who help RSI sufferers will find in this book new and useful concepts and hands-on techniques that can benefit their patients. While most of the presentation will be phrased for the layman, we've made every effort to make it readable by all.

What Is RSI?

RSI in our context is muscle pain or nerve problems of the hands, arms, or shoulders—what doctors call *the upper extremity*—believed to be caused by overuse. It can also include the neck and back, and may be accompanied by burning, numbness, tingling, or pins-and-needles sensations. The symptoms range from dull and diffuse aching to intense, searing, and very specific pain. You may even be unable to use your hands or you may have difficulty with coordination.

In the 1980's, the computer became America's favorite toy. Soon it was being used with passion and obsession, and with incessant, static posture at workstations that had little or no anatomical consideration given to them. And so entered the disorder of the 90's, RSI, the most complicated and controversial problem of the workplace. RSI is a perplexing mystery because it adds up so slowly that the body has plenty of time to adapt and compensate. This enables the body to protect itself from symptoms, but essentially hides RSI from you while you fall under its spell! When you finally notice symptoms, it is as if a switch were suddenly turned on, despite the fact that the problems probably have been building for as long as two years, perhaps much more.

As you might imagine, the earlier it is diagnosed, the easier it is to treat and the more rapid your recovery. But its onset is so sneaky, and you are so scared to admit that it is happening, that early intervention is not the norm. Many people ignore it until it becomes serious. In all but the most severe cases, however, improvement can be expected with the proper treatment.

RSI is a soft tissue disease, meaning it affects muscles and nerves, but over time it can also affect bones and joints, or cause other "systemic" problems. For instance, you might develop problems with the gastrointestinal system, circulation, or central nervous system. Essentially, it is an "overuse" syndrome where a constant, repetitive, or forceful activity causes the damage. To give you an idea how controversial it is, some theorists even dispute the significance of repetition as a contributing factor. They argue that posture, ergonomics, and health explain it all. By their reckoning, could we all sit at a computer for a 45-year, 50-hour-per-week career with no ill effects? We're doubtful.

But why is RSI so much more of a problem now than in the days of typewriters and "typing pools," in which office workers routinely pounded out reams of business letters all day long? First, repetitive strain injuries didn't originate with computers—they've been a fact of life in all sorts of careers from butcher to baker to typist. If the number of reported cases was smaller in the past, one explanation might be the balance of power; in the past, people tolerated work injuries as if they were unavoidable. Now we have more protection for work-induced injury, and more priority is placed on curing the disease instead of sweeping it under the carpet. But the more important factor is the work itself. RSI wasn't as much of a problem with typewriters because typewriters had steeply stepped rows of keys, requiring you to hold your hands up. This meant that you couldn't rest your arms on the work surface, so there were no pinch points. There was also a lot more variety of motion using a typewriter, correcting mistakes, rolling the platen back-and-forth with one hand, swinging the carriage return lever with the other hand, and changing paper. These factors combined to provide a lot more exercise—invigoration is the best word—for your arms than you get using today's "efficient" computer keyboard. Lastly, even employees in a typing pool probably didn't type all day long, let alone with their hands in one position, but we do now.

The Public Cost   Estimates of the total cost of RSI are staggering and rising, ranging from $7 - $20 billion per year in the U.S alone. There are hundreds of thousands of workers' compensation claims each year, averaging over $20,000 each and with the increasing specialization and computerization of the industrial workforce, the numbers show no sign of abatement. But if you're reading this book for your own health, the statistics and public cost are probably of no concern to you, so we won't belabor them. Instead, you are concerned about your own health and livelihood. The only statistic that matters is *one*. What will be a concern along the way toward resolving your problem, however, is the attitude of those around you.

The Public Misperception   Until you yourself experience the pain of RSI and the waves of confusion, frustration, and fear that accompany an injury that has no *event* clearly associated with it, you too will probably be one of the folks compounding the misperception. But don't feel bad—I [JB] still understood very little about RSI until a year after being operated upon! Perhaps I even propagated as much misinformation as the next guy. The unfortunate situation is that there are extremely few facts—substantiated cause-and-effect data—in this field, so misinformation is the norm. The best we have is what's called *anecdotal information*—the stories of individuals—and the insights of observers based on their involvement with patients.

> "I was accused of psychological problems, and treated like the enemy by my company, for whom I had worked like a demon."
>
> -- Patient A

Carpal Tunnel Syndrome   The first point of widespread confusion is mistaking carpal tunnel syndrome for all RSI. Debunking that myth will be one of our most emphatic themes. We will show that true carpal tunnel syndrome, in which the actual cause of the problem is confined to the wrist area, is fairly rare. For most computer users, the cause of the problem is much more widespread, involving aggravation points up and down the neck, shoulder, and arm. Attempts to address only the wrist area are almost always followed in a matter of months by a litany of other symptoms. You can imagine how depressing this is after you've had surgery on the wrists as some of our case study patients have. If you don't have a really strong constitution this can be a very tough time to get through without showing outward signs of defeat or surrendering altogether.

The Malingerer Myth The next misperception is that RSI sufferers are slackers, whereas in our experience, the opposite is true—many RSI sufferers quite literally work their fingers to the bone.

> "Once I became a workers' compensation case I found that many people were biased in that they feel all injured workers are simply trying to get out of work and that they are lazy and dishonest. I encountered this prejudice at work, with the insurance people, and in the medical profession."
>
> -- Patient D.

Adding to the confusion and mismanagement, the insurance companies are often part of the problem, not the cure. We won't delve too deeply into the legal side of the RSI dilemma, but in his article, "Twenty Clinical Truths About RSI," Peter Bower, M.D., sums it up pretty well: "Insurance companies are uniformly ignorant, or obstructionist, or both, when it comes to treating these problems."

> "Dealing with the insurance carrier and the workers' compensation liaison at work was always difficult, I never felt that they had my best interest in mind."
>
> -- Patient D.

References

Twenty Clinical Truths About RSI, Peter Bower, M.D, June 1994
http://www.tifaq.com/articles/20_rsi_truths.html

The Importance of Early Identification

Because RSI is almost certainly both cumulative and the result of repetitive actions, the passage of time is a key factor in the progression of the disorder. Consequently, early intervention is crucial. Although it is very difficult for individuals with new, minor symptoms to appreciate this point, every "sob story" of chronic RSI on the various Internet discussion groups drives this point home:

Address your symptoms when they first arise!

Stop or reduce your work as best you can. Although a strict correlation between delaying treatment and its effect on rehabilitation time is impossible to establish, we will suggest a rule of thumb, based on our experiences: for every week that you work with RSI symptoms, add one month to the time it will take you to heal.

RSI in computer users creates a repeating cycle of pain and injury that "snowballs" somewhat secretively through all the parts of the upper extremity, and is rarely identified properly, let alone early. For instance, many patients will notice something that seems like an odd ache or pain and naturally want to believe it is just that... a sore muscle. They hope that some rest will make it heal, like every other injury they've ever had. And the worst part of RSI is that in the early stages it often does! They rest the part that hurts, and sometimes shift the load to another part. One way or another, the quick cure gives them enough confidence to believe the problem *was* incidental and isolated, not chronic, cumulative, and systemic. Some weeks or months later, they have another, perhaps different symptom. This is how the injury-pain-injury cycle starts, making this problem so damaging. It also demonstrates the denial-delay cycle that makes it so difficult to catch early.

> "I did not seek help immediately. I waited until my hands were too cramped to move after five months of 45-60 hour weeks of nonstop typing."
>
> -- Patient A.

If you catch it early, your rehab may consist simply of strengthening, stretching, and some work habit changes. Once you cross the line where you've got substantial muscle inflammation—you won't always feel it—or nerve sensation changes, you've missed your chance for early intervention.

You may need lots of hands-on help from a still-rare breed of therapist who knows this condition most literally inside-out. Nonetheless, our experience indicates that even the most severely injured can get substantial relief.

Prevention Is the Key

Better than early identification and intervention is prevention. If you are responsible for a workplace full of computer users, start a training program. Make good ergonomics the norm, not the exception. Encourage early reporting of problems. But most importantly, foster an environment of authentic caring, balance between work and other activities, and genuine problem solving, not quick fixes or simply "compliance." Compliance implies an attempt to satisfy regulatory requirements or insurance companies with little regard for people and their health.

Prevention is not an easy road, or necessarily an encouraging one. It's entirely possible that many individuals can afford to break all of the ergonomic and common sense rules. Some can afford to work in poor postures indefinitely, perhaps because their bodies are young and resilient, or simply not susceptible to the tension that causes RSI. And others just won't heed any warnings until damage occurs. A reasonable approach to take is to focus on sending out good information, establishing an atmosphere of vigilance about the health risk, and mostly, doing everything possible to encourage early detection and intervention. This will be the focus of our final section.

There is a Solution

Contrary to frequent references you may read suggesting that you are condemned to a lifetime of suffering, our experience is that most RSI cases can improve. We don't have wild stories of one-hour cures where a few simple tricks cure you. After all, by our account, if you have a serious RSI problem, it took you several years to cause the problem. So it won't be cured in hours, or even days.

How long should recovery from chronic RSI take? Haven't we come to expect modern medicine to provide a quick cure even for a problem that was years in the making? Maybe. But this injury is related to muscle vitality and nerve health. If a quick fix is available, it's not well publicized. You may read or hear about some therapies that claim almost instantaneous improvement. Ours does not. But neither does it take as long as it took you to cause the damage. Your body probably waged war against RSI's mistreatment for years before surrendering and fighting back with fatigue, inflammation, and pain. But the body does have an incredible capacity for rejuvenation, if given the proper chance. Rarely are nerves truly damaged, but they do heal slowly. Rarer still would it be to find muscles that are unable to return to their normal vitality. Muscles are routinely in a state of build-up and breakdown, so they heal very agreeably if you treat them nicely.

But we talk in terms of *healing from RSI*, rather than being *cured*. If you've been typing for years, and you intend to keep working at the keyboard, we do believe you will remain susceptible to repeated damage. The best description we've heard is that your nerves will be "fragile." Consequently, you must make enough changes to your work habits that you no longer accumulate damage more quickly than you dissipate its effects.

It's Not Your Fault

The question of fault frequently arises about RSI. It's common to come across statements like this:

> *"... anyone suffering from chronic pain will have trigger points*,*
> *due either to their lack of exercise or bad posture."*

While exercise and posture are important factors and will be involved in our theory, poor posture, by our account, is a result, not a cause. As far as exercise, we frequently see very active people with RSI; they are simply behind the keyboard too long, and too tenaciously. The history of serious RSI patients is riddled with people whose symptoms were unable to be explained by doctors. These patients frequently tell stories of being labeled psychosomatic, hypochondriac, or manic-depressive.

---

* Trigger points are tender spots in muscle or nerve, causing pain at another location. Much more on trigger points, later.

> "At one point, I was questioned whether there was an inordinate amount of stress that may be causing my symptoms. Were there personal problems I was having that would need to be discussed with a counselor? In other words, was I imagining what I was feeling or better yet, was I crazy?"
>
> -- Patient B.

We will certainly concur that there is a mind-body connection at play in RSI, but the problems don't arise in the brain. For hard-core computer users, they arise in a work ethic or compulsion combined with many physical circumstances—and countless millions of repetitions over many years—to undermine the body's inherent vitality. It's not because you are weak, or unsuited to the work, or unfit. *It's not your fault.*

Understanding the Traditional Medical Response

The traditional medical community is only beginning to comprehend and cope with computer-related RSI. Unlike the impressive record of accomplishment to which we have become accustomed with systemic problems like the gastrointestinal system or very event-specific problems such as broken bones, RSI presents a far different challenge. Certainly, physicians and surgeons have many successful RSI recoveries to their credit. But the *range* of results runs the gamut from quick recoveries to abysmal failure, sometimes with insult added to injury, as patients have been advised to seek psychiatric help.

We will not bombard you with the statistics on success/failure rates for patients who have had carpal tunnel surgery. If the rates for surgical resolution of RSI were high enough, you wouldn't be reading this book... it wouldn't even exist. But why is there such a questionable record?

First, the surgery is often mis-directed, mistaking effects for causes. Symptoms of RSI often occur in an area downstream, with respect to the nerve, from the problem spot. For instance, in our clinical experience, true cases of carpal tunnel syndrome are rare, but the surgery is fairly common. There may have been as many as half a million carpal tunnel surgeries performed in the U.S. last year alone! When you have wrist or hand pain, the cause might not be in your wrist, but very possibly your chest, an area called the thoracic outlet. That was the experience of one of our case study patients who had unsuccessful bilateral (both wrists) carpal tunnel surgery.

Second, again with respect to surgery, it usually focuses on too narrow of a solution. For instance, even if the ulnar nerve has been diagnosed with damage in the vicinity of your elbow, resolving that one spot surgically— the nerve can be moved out of harm's way—does not address the larger situation. The nerve could have been trapped by fibrous tissue that builds up from years of working in one position, or healing could be prevented by reduced blood flow due to muscle tension.

Even the non-surgical treatments offered by conventional practitioners do not have a great track record. The almost universal response of M.D.s when an RSI patient first "presents," is to recommend a wrist brace and anti-inflammatory drugs. One is a crutch, the other a palliative. If you've been typing a relatively short amount of time (less than two years) perhaps this approach is not entirely unadvisable... at least it's non-invasive (although you might not agree after you feel the way the anti-inflammatory drugs attack your stomach lining). We won't get too deep into the therapy right now, but for serious RSI sufferers, crutches will prevent the real solution you need: reconditioning your muscles for strength and stamina. Palliatives might make the pain go away for a short amount of time, but they don't stop the circumstances that cause the pain.

> **What did your doctors prescribe?**
>
> "Anti-inflammatories, cortisone, narcotic painkillers, anti-depressants, Percocett, Duract, Nuerontin, Elavil, Utram, Advil, Aleve."
>
> -- Patient C.

Is there a common denominator to the traditional treatments? Absolutely. First, American medicine is fixated on structural problems and solutions. In other words, most problems are treated as if they are a broken bone or a ruptured appendix. Using an age-old analogy, if all you have is a hammer, everything looks like a nail. This fixation means that we try to fix everything with physical devices or remedies, using tools to change the structure of the body. This misses or downplays the notion that nature is a *process*, not just a structure. It consists of relationships and forces in equilibrium. If you can understand and work with the processes, the remedy will be more successful. Without going too far off into extreme alternative medicine, consider simple nearsightedness. We've perfected the art of making eyeglasses, but has any mainstream effort been directed to the possible solution of strengthening the eye muscles to achieve better focus?

No, our medical direction is overwhelmingly inclined to solving problems with devices and structural solutions.

In the excellent introduction to *The Alternative Medicine Yellow Pages*, several aspects of the medical culture are also cited as contributing to the weaknesses of the traditional response. First, medical schools are organized around organs; each department teaches about one system or another, so a problem like RSI that combines several systems has no sponsor and therefore, no proponents. Second, today's financial structure in medicine encourages quick fixes and has little accommodation for root cause analysis and resolution. The reimbursement system has no means whatsoever for compensating cures that cross over various disciplines or passages of time. Even the billing identification system bears this out, as all treatment is classified by existing conditions. Even the legal environment fosters a predisposition to the status quo, since malpractice is judged not by how effective or logical a solution is, but by how consistent the service is with existing practice.

> "I was perplexed and somewhat disturbed to see that my visit to my family doctor, to discuss my worn down ulnar nerve and its transient numbness, pain, and pinching sensation, was classified on the bill as Palsy, Other."
>
> -- Patient E.

A final reason for the traditional response is lack of sufficient information. Better information is only recently starting to accumulate on therapeutic solutions to RSI. Increasingly doctors are learning which techniques have been successful with ergonomics, muscular therapies, and relief of nerve entrapment problems. By the collective judgment of the medical community as a whole, the solution appears very much in debate, but we believe we are zero-ing in on the solution.

> "My doctor had me take a blood test to check for arthritis and Lyme disease."
>
> -- Patient A.

References

The Alternative Medicine Yellow Pages
http://www.amazon.com or your local library
Future Medicine Publishing Company
Tiburon, CA 94920

Our Springboard: The Existing Literature

If you go to AMAZON.COM and search for *RSI* and *ergonomics*, you'll find much of what the world knows about RSI, in book form. There's a lot of great information, and as you might guess, a lot of drivel. A fair amount of the information in our book can be found in existing literature. The challenge is separating the good from the bad and deciding where and how it applies. Then there's the portion we've added in the form of new ideas and new ways of regarding some of the existing information.

Consider the following four sources, which comprise a good cross-section of the RSI thought bank:

Repetitive Strain Injury: A Computer User's Guide
By Dr. Emil Pascarelli & Deborah Quilter, 1994

This is the leading work on RSI, with an almost encyclopedic coverage of the topic. Pascarelli presents a good case for drawing a link between the general scenario of computer/environmental conditions and the physiological conditions that result. It is the basis for pursuing neuromuscular therapy and has paved the way for the therapy offered by many practitioners, Suparna Damany among them. Suparna collaborated with Dr. Pascarelli and developed her therapeutic approach from his foundation. In this landmark work, Pascarelli dissects every fiber of the RSI fabric, leaving only the actual diagnosis to the practitioners. We will take this foundation one step further by identifying a specific therapeutic strategy that addresses common denominators among chronic, computer-related RSI sufferers.

> "I think the Pascarelli book described it [my condition], but I was too far-gone to help myself."
>
> -- Patient A.

The Natural Treatment of Carpal Tunnel Syndrome: How to Treat 'Computer Wrist' Without Surgery
By Ray C. Wunderlich, Jr., M.D. , 1993

This 50-page brochure is a wonderfully concise exposé on a wide range of contributing factors and potential therapies, almost a taxonomy of the RSI world. For instance, it lists causes as diverse as nutrition, and hyperthyroidism, and therapies from reflexology (foot manipulation) to surgery. At four dollars, it is definitely the most "bang for the buck." If you're inclined toward hypochondria, you may think after reading it that you have the plague. However, Wunderlich makes few judgment calls—he just spells out options. The one he does seem to harp on is nutrition. In his intro and conclusion he suggests that RSI is the culmination of technology and Twinkies (our words, not his). As a broccoli eating, exercycling, computer professional, I found this offensive. Nonetheless, you must get this booklet and read it in case your RSI is actually caused by the plague. Our lawyers insist.

Carpal Tunnel Syndrome And Repetitive Stress Injuries: The Comprehensive Guide to Prevention, Treatment, & Recovery
By Tammy Crouch, 1995

Similar to Wunderlich in that it presents everything under the sun, this one is from the patient's perspective, and more detailed, at 150 pages. As with Wunderlich, you will come away with your head spinning, unsure whether anyone has any idea what's going on. Note however that this book is from 1995 and was a trailblazer in a land that at the time resembled the Sahara desert. It collects more practical RSI information in one place than perhaps any other source, and it's written from an RSI patient's perspective. What it doesn't attempt to offer is decision making... diagnostic advice. We will take up where it leaves off.

End Your Carpal Tunnel Pain Without Surgery
By Kate Montgomery, 1998

This book presents a 12-step therapeutic course that offers very specific exercises but, we believe, stops just short of defining the scenario that confronts the computer user with serious RSI problems. If your problems have just started, and they are typical computer-related RSI, this book is definitely an excellent source and may as it claims, solve your problems in minutes. But if your situation is chronic, this book will not give you what we believe is a clear picture of the specific forces tearing you apart, and might leave you unprepared for the long haul. Simply put, it is more generalized than what we will present. For instance, among the ten or so therapies that Montgomery describes, she talks about neuromuscular massage and trigger points without many specifics. You can get the impression that you might resolve a muscle spasm by massaging it for five minutes, but our case study patients have required repeated sessions of vigorous massage to resolve some problems. We will zero-in on this therapy and identify the individual spots based on hundreds of computer users. We'll describe what the therapist feels as the trigger points resolve, and lay out in detail the entire range of trauma up and down the arm.

Our Alternative

Our intention is that this book will actually be usable as a guide for the layman to manage his own healing process and for therapists to perform hands-on work. If you find that your situation matches the picture we paint, we encourage you to find a therapist who will apply the program in this book. Don't be embarrassed to actually give them a copy. The state of knowledge in this area is so new and disjointed that it's both astounding and perplexing. For instance, in Wunderlich's $4 booklet, buried in the obscure references to reflexology, is a sentence that described exactly the symptom that explained how I got relief from three years of discomfort:

> *"Stansbery has found that virtually every single patient had this trigger point on the inside of the elbow. He works it for two months and they go back to work."*

My jaw dropped open when I read that an obscure practitioner had routine experiences with a therapy of which my surgeon was completely unaware… a therapy that Suparna had performed on me to solve what his surgery did not. That is the state of knowledge on this topic… a state we hope to improve.

> "Nothing [in the literature] described my situation that allowed me to say 'That's what I have.'"
>
> -- Patient B.

And what will our contribution consist of, the added portion alluded to earlier?

- ❑ We will spell out what we believe is a general syndrome that explains most computer-related RSI.

- ❑ Unlike the existing literature, which is either very multi-purpose or non-committal, we *will* make the judgment call. We propose to know what your problem is, or at least the specific set of problems from which you must choose. Yes, we will have to generalize to do this, so we leave it up to you to determine if you fit the generalization.

- ❑ We will assume your problem is not bad nutrition, hyperthyroidism, or pregnancy. It's not, is it? Perhaps the most repeated trivial factor mentioned throughout the literature is that pregnancy causes fluid retention and can aggravate the median nerve.

- ❑ We will discount (but not completely disregard) the way you hold the telephone in your neck, and other incidental factors. Many poor work habits can certainly contribute to problems, but our concentration will be on hard-core computer use. Be forewarned, though, that posture is *not* incidental. We will wave our finger at you like your mother and say, "sit up straight."

- ❑ We will distinguish causes from symptoms, one of the most difficult aspects of sorting out this mystery.

- ❑ We will describe how to get relief, with specific therapies, including some techniques you can do yourself, and others that are more effective with a therapist.

- ❑ We'll spell out how to improve and correct your way of working, including workstation ergonomics and new rules for using your body.

- ❑ Finally we'll provide very specific, *actionable* items that can be used to implement an RSI prevention program.

Our Theory In A Nutshell

RSI is caused by working in an extremely repetitive fashion, in one position, for years. Your muscles lock up in that position and fatigue, causing your posture to collapse forward. The unnaturally tensed muscles get inflamed and frequently pinch your nerves and blood vessels. Your body lays down fibrous tissue to accommodate the fixed posture, tethering nerves in place and causing excessive wear and tear on them. The constant repetition, contorted positions, and small range of motion cause tendons to get sticky and inflamed, causing irritation and fluid buildup. All of these changes reduce circulation and overwhelm what would normally be the body's ongoing recuperative process.

If you treat individual sore spots instead of the whole superstructure of the arm, the symptoms will move from one spot to another. Instead, you must recondition the entire upper extremity, and the way you work, including workload, posture, ergonomics, strength, stamina, flexibility, and overall health.

To understand why this all happens, we present the number one physiological truth of RSI: muscles, tendons, and bones (collectively the musculoskeletal system) will adapt somewhat to almost any habitual posture and activity. Unfortunately, they will do this with no regard or accommodation whatsoever to the nervous system, which has no such adaptability. Your nerves may be the messengers of the deteriorating state of affairs, or the actual recipients of the damage.

We'll spell this out in excruciating detail in our upcoming section on theory.

Our Case Study Patients

You've already read some of the comments from and about our case study patients. We'll include more of these comments as we go along, to show how their experiences not only support our ideas but have been the inspiration for many of them. These patients represent a small sampling of the patients Suparna has treated, and are typical of the results she's achieved. The following summaries will introduce their entire stories, so you can understand their situations.

These patients' collective experiences are very possibly the most significant fact-finding information any of us are likely to encounter in RSI. It's conceivable that controlled scientific studies will never substantiate much RSI theory because of the length of time that it takes to cause RSI. Reproducing the actual scenarios in voluntary laboratory situations is difficult and unlikely.

Patient A, "Alison"

Alison had been programming for eleven years when she noticed her right hand going numb while using the mouse. A coworker suggested switching to the other hand. She switched for two weeks and then switched back, no longer having any pain in the original hand. She was working non-stop on a very stressful project that had tight deadlines and a lot of overtime. She began to notice that her upper back and neck were sore all the time, even lying down. Then she noticed her hands felt tired when driving. Soon she wasn't able to grip things. Both of her hands started going numb at night. One day her hands just cramped up and she could not relax them. Her hands and forearms began to ache 'round-the-clock.

She did not seek help immediately, but waited until after more than five months of 45-60 hour weeks of nonstop typing, until her hands were too cramped to move. Alison's experience at the hands of the traditional medical community is somewhat of an epic adventure. The first doctor she went to said she had tendinitis (inflammation of the tendons that bend the fingers). He said to cut back to 40 hours a week. (How's that for "advice for the modern worker!") He prescribed the usual first attempt of wrist braces and painkillers, neither of which helped. After wasting many weeks with this sort of guesswork, she realized that this doctor was not having much luck, so she went to another doctor that was recommended by someone she worked with. She was in so much pain that she didn't have to wait the usual eight weeks required of new patients. It was already three months since she first went to see a doctor and she had no relief from her symptoms. This doctor ordered an electromyogram (an electrical muscle/nerve test). The results showed that she had bilateral carpal tunnel syndrome. By this time, she was in so much pain, that he said she should not type. This meant that she could not work, so she went out on medical leave.

The doctor tried cortisone shots and then said her only option was surgery. She got a second opinion, and eventually had surgery on both wrists. The numbness and tingling went away immediately after surgery. (Readers, remember this subtle fact: *the symptoms went away.*) She went to rehabilitation and eventually, they started her typing again. Unfortunately, her hands started going numb again within a week of typing! Her hands would also go numb whenever she lifted her arms up to her shoulders.

At this point, she tried a myofascial therapist (a massage specialist that focuses on muscle and connective tissue) and a chiropractor, without consistent results. She felt better after the myofascial therapy sessions, but it was not helping her get back to working condition. Her employer brought her back to work at a job that did not require typing. Her body hurt, even using a voice dictation system. Her doctors ran other tests to no avail. Her employer began to get impatient. They considered firing her, because the insurance company informed them that she should have been better three months after surgery.

Then, through a coworker, she found her way to Suparna, who convinced Alison's employer, her doctor, and the insurance company that she had thoracic outlet syndrome, complicated by other repetitive strain factors. She was treated by Suparna three times a week and finally could see some progress. After substantial therapy, she eventually started back at work two hours a day for two weeks and then increased to four hours a day. After two more weeks she increased again to six hours a day. She's since increased to eight hours a day and has only minor symptoms.

Patient B, "Beth"

Beth had been typing for eleven years when she noticed symptoms that included nagging pain in the right thumb, forearm, and elbow. Over the course of three years the symptoms came and went, moving around, but finally settling in the upper torso. Doctors suspected tendinitis, tennis elbow, myofascial pain, high stress levels, and ultimately her mental soundness. She was prescribed large dosages of Ibuprofen and then anti-inflammatory drugs and a cursory attempt at physical therapy, all to no avail.

After several episodes, an acquaintance referred her to Suparna. It took four months of rigorous physical therapy, including deep tissue massage to break up muscle spasms throughout the chest, and a regimen of stretching and strengthening exercises, but she's back at work. The biggest physical change in her workstation is a simple keyboard tray. More importantly, she practices other techniques such as emphasizing large muscle movements instead of bending her wrist, and maintaining a more balanced posture.

Patient C, "Chris"

Chris had been typing for 14 years, and had a wide range of symptoms: left arm atrophy, numbness, coldness, and tingling, from shoulder to fingers; pain in the chest, back, and neck; and intermittent pain in the left wrist. Along the therapeutic trail, doctors prescribed cortisone shots and a veritable smorgasbord of drugs without results.

Suparna employed every weapon in her arsenal, including deep massage, extensive work on the thoracic outlet, ergonomic changes, and physical fitness rehabilitation. But the success of Suparna's treatment was only partial—Chris estimates 50-65%. However, Chris did eventually get additional relief from another therapy, one based on the concept that low oxygen supply to the muscles and nerves is to blame. This theory has its roots in behavior modification, and we'll explain more about it in our discussion of therapy. We specifically include this patient's experience because it's instructive for the perspective it adds. First, even the partial success with our techniques is actually reassuring, in view of the severity of Chris's symptoms. Beyond that, it helps reinforce that ours is no magic cure-all—patients do have problems that arise from other sources, and other answers are out there, perhaps for you too.

Patient D, "Drew"

Drew had been typing for six years when symptoms first occurred, but they turned very serious after nine years, especially with the change from a terminal to a PC and mouse. Drew's symptoms included pain, achiness, and extreme tightness from the fingers all the way up to the back. At times, it also caused headaches. At its worst, there was also loss of the fine motor skills in the hands, and reduced range of motion in the neck.

One doctor prescribed Advil and splints. Another used a nerve conduction test that ruled out carpal tunnel syndrome. A luxurious four-minute exam (!) by an orthopedist resulted in a prescription for the anti-inflammatory drug, Relafen. After determining that the Relafen did not work, he suspected rheumatoid arthritis or lupus and referred Drew to a rheumatologist. The rheumatologist's examination showed no indication of arthritis, so he diagnosed "overuse syndrome" and summarily sentenced Drew to a regimen of physical therapy called "work hardening." This apparently is modern medicine's version of being exiled to Siberia. This made Drew's pain much worse.

Finally, Drew came upon Dr. Emil Pascarelli and Suparna and the rehabilitation truly began. With a detailed diagnosis from Dr. Pascarelli and *extensive* hands-on treatment and ergonomic help from Suparna, Drew is back at work full time. Like many serious RSI sufferers, Drew's symptoms are not eradicated... they are controlled. The controls include better work habits, stretching, breaks, an emphasis on balanced posture, relaxation, and more techniques that we will describe in detail.

Patient E, "Edward"

Edward developed symptoms after 13 years while working on what he described as his "typically maniacal" programming project. First, he would awake at night with his hand numb. Then tightness and aching in the fingers were noticeable when typing. This became numbness after a while, the most ominous of RSI symptoms because it is a precursor to motor damage—the inability of the nerve to operate your limbs.

His general practitioner prescribed an anti-inflammatory (which gave him ulcer-like stomach symptoms) and a wrist brace for use at night. Neither seemed to give conclusive results, but the symptoms weren't terribly aggravating, so he persevered for a year. At that time, his employer referred him to an orthopedic hand specialist who conducted a nerve test that indicated damage of a nerve that passes around the elbow. After persevering for another year, he took the surgeon's recommendation to move the nerve away from the damaging elbow joint. Immediately after the surgery and for a few months Edward was good-as-new, but in six months' time the symptoms returned, identical to before the surgery.

Edward came under Suparna's care when she started an RSI prevention program at his workplace. Suparna subsequently found considerable deposits of tissue binding his nerve in the upper arm, and resolved these by massaging them out over the course of several weeks. That treatment, along with her regimen of exercises, stretching, and new work habits has enabled Edward to control his symptoms and work relatively pain free.

Patient F, "Frank"

Our last case study patient is a simple success story, no parade of erroneous diagnoses, and no drugs or surgery, just well-conceived therapy. Despite its simplicity, it's an especially valuable story because it reinforces the point that addressing symptoms early—with the right therapy—will remedy a relatively serious RSI situation.

Frank had been typing for over ten years as a software developer and tester when he started to have severe pain in the pad of his thumb. Unlike our other case study patients, Frank sought help within weeks of noticing symptoms… because Suparna was seeing patients at his workplace at the time. She showed him that his hand was just one of many sore areas; his arm, neck, and shoulder blade had several intense sore spots that he hardly noticed, but were surprisingly tender to the touch. It turns out that he was aware of other aches and pains, those in the shoulder and neck, but had been dismissing them as unrelated to work, just something to try to ignore. Suparna observed that his seated posture was collapsed far forward, and as is often the case, he had severe muscle imbalance because of this: the front of his chest was overly tense, and his shoulder blade area was very weak.

Throughout the remainder of the book, you'll read how our techniques— massage, joint mobilization, strengthening, stretching, better work habits, and ergonomics—helped Frank heal in weeks, prevented him from becoming a chronic sufferer, and enabled him to work without pain.

Part 2: Theory

How Computer Users Get RSI

In this section, we'll explain the causes of computer-related RSI and the logic behind the recommendations that we will make in our discussion of therapy. Along the way, we'll describe the anatomy that's involved, symptoms, predisposing factors, diagnosis, and prognosis.

One of the most frustrating things you'll notice about the entire RSI subject is the abundance of people with information and advice, but absolutely no substantiation behind it. For instance, many folks are fond of suggesting that you should work with your forearms parallel to the ground and your elbows at a 90-degree angle. But how does a 90-degree angle help someone who has been told that his or her ulnar nerve has been worn down where it goes around the elbow? Wouldn't a more relaxed angle cause less wear? The answer is no one knows. There are no "controlled studies," where all other variables are eliminated. And there are unlikely to be any. That's the difference between this soft tissue disease and others. And that's the challenge I made to Suparna when she presented herself as yet another theorist in the vast sea of the unsubstantiated. Why should I believe her any more than the hundreds who preceded her? The answer is that she has a significant track record of patients she's helped. The following pages detail the theory that explains how those patients sustained their injuries and how they found the path to recovery.

The RSI Scenario, Step-By-Step

If you're well into the RSI world and have read all of the literature, we should forewarn you that you won't find any miraculous new revelations here... well, maybe just a few. What you will find though is a substantive, sensible, and very specific model that puts the information together to explain most computer-related problems.

Let's start with an analogy, albeit an extreme one. Imagine you've been hanging upside-down, eight hours a day for ten years... and you've been holding your arms out straight in front of you while hanging around. How do think your ankles will feel after seven or eight years? What sort of sensation do you think your toes will be capable of? How 'bout if I told you, as your medical professional, that to repair the damage, I prescribe better nutrition and more sleep—you have a horrible lifestyle. We better have you try braces on your ankles to keep them from stretching too much. Oh yes, and vitamin B6, lots of it. Acupuncture, homeopathic drugs, and electromagnets for the pain, gut-wrenching anti-inflammatories for the swelling, and if all else fails, surgery to separate that heavy torso from those poor feet. As silly as it sounds, these are some of the typical recommendations from the medical community. Get the point? Even if you believe our exaggerated analogy is only slightly applicable, it still presents the basis for our case. Namely, you must stop being distracted by quick fixes and get busy directly attacking the stresses on your system.

Here's how we think it works when you're right-side up:

❏ Computer-related RSI is caused by working, often compulsively, in a single, hands-suspended posture for a long, long time.

❏ All of the muscles that hold up your head, shoulders, and arms go into a state of constant tension called "spasm." They eventually fatigue, and lose their strength and stamina. Your body does so many things to compensate that you don't feel most of these sensations until years have passed and damage starts to occur.

❏ If stress and complex psychological factors are contributing to your condition, you may also be cheating your muscles of oxygen by unnecessarily and imperceptibly tensing your whole upper extremity. This is one of the most variable and immeasurable components of RSI, but a likely multiplying factor, meaning it will exacerbate all of the factors that follow.

❏ As your neck and shoulders fatigue, particularly your shoulder blade muscles, your shoulders roll forward... you slouch. Instead of a balanced posture with minimal tension, you are out of balance, and it takes constant effort to hold yourself up. All of the literature agrees on this much. This persistent slouch causes the neck and chest muscles to tighten up while the shoulder blade muscles get stretched out.

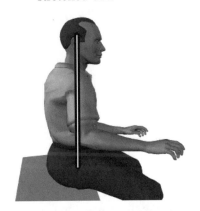

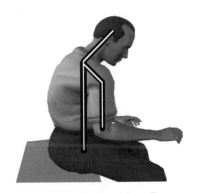

Low Stress, Balanced Posture

In a balanced position, your back and shoulder muscles don't have to work so hard.

High Stress, Slouching Posture

When you lean forward, your chest and neck muscles pinch off nerves and blood supply.

❏ What doesn't come out clearly in the literature is the result: your front neck muscles tug on the area where the nerves and blood vessels to your arms pass out between the first rib and collarbone, an area called the thoracic outlet. Your shoulders also collapse over your armpit, pressing on a concentrated intersection of nerves called the brachial plexus, which gives rise to all the nerves of the arm. Pressure on the nerves causes a variety of symptoms in the arms, including pain, tingling, and numbness. Pressure on the blood vessel reduces blood flow to the arm, inhibiting the healing process and removal of the waste products of muscle metabolism. In some cases, the pectoralis minor muscle from the chest to the arm becomes hypertrophied (thickened) and pinches off a small gap through which nerves and blood vessels pass.

❏ Your body begins an elaborate, invisible pattern of compensation called the pain cycle. Overworked muscles become inflamed, which is initially a healthy, healing mechanism. You avoid these muscles, adjust your posture unnaturally to compensate, and eventually overload other previously uninvolved muscles. The inflamed muscles often cut off nerves and blood flow because your body was not designed for them to be in constant tension. In several places up and down the arm, the nerves and blood vessels weave their way right between muscle, tendon, and bone. You rest at night but go back to work the next morning, before the healing process is complete, so the metabolic waste products build up in your arm, compounding the inflammation.

❑   The fatigue of the large neck and shoulder muscles, causes the forearm and hand muscles to overwork. Even without this overloading phenomenon, the action of typing taxes the small bands of muscles that drive the fingers. These muscles are more prone to the tension/fatigue cycle than larger ones. If you're obsessed with working as proficiently as possible, you may also make extreme contortions that stress these small muscles to the utmost. One example is holding the left Control key with your left thumb while pressing the Esc key with your left middle finger (a common hot-key in the old Windows 3.x). Actions like this cause the maximum possible irritation in the forearm, wrist, and hand. Some practitioners believe that these irritating motions cause the tendon sheaths in the carpal tunnel to become sticky and resistant to smoothly gliding. If a medical exam considers only the circumstances at the wrist, a diagnosis of tendinitis, tenosynovitis (inflammation of the lubricating membrane around a tendon), or even arthritis is commonplace but fails to address the big picture.

❑   The most flagrant of typing offenses, cited by all RSI theorists, are bending the wrist up (dorsiflexion), and bending it out (ulnar deviation). These positions overwork the small muscle bands of the forearm as you reach with the fingertips instead of moving the whole arm. If you work to the point of inflammation in the forearm, the resultant swelling can cause fluid buildup in the wrist. This in turn could easily be labeled, solely in terms of symptoms, as carpal tunnel syndrome, again with no attention to the root cause.

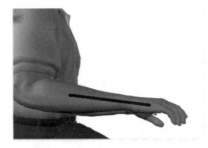

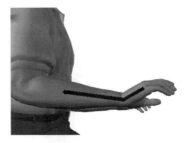

Correct, "Neutral" Wrist Position

In a straight line, the tendons going through your wrist are relatively free from friction.

Dorsiflexion

Bending the wrist causes friction at the tendon sheaths and can reduce blood flow.

❑ As you lose stamina, you may rest your hands on the work surfaces more. Pressure on the wrist can cause reduced blood flow and further pinch the median nerve going to the fingers. The nerve or blood vessel going to the two smallest fingers can also become pinched in a small passageway in the pad of the hand, called Guyon's Canal, resulting in another syndrome, named for the canal.

❑ Let's take a closer look at muscle spasms, those knots of muscle in continuous tension. Note that these are different from muscles that are cramped. In a cramp, the muscle suddenly, quite agonizingly contracts. Muscle spasms, however, become sore and inflamed, *but rarely do you even feel these tender spots* unless a trained therapist palpates deeply to show you how different they feel than your other healthy muscles.

❑ Some practitioners have promoted the idea that the muscles take on the qualities of ligaments, laying down fibrous tissue because they are bearing a static load. If, as an RSI sufferer, you've ever noticed that your arms were feeling very wiry or taut, this is likely what you've felt.

❑ One particular small muscle action is the pronation of the hands, turning the thumbs down to meet the keyboard. This action alone may account for the most universal, acute symptom noted in the anecdotal literature, called a nerve "trigger point" near the inside of the elbow. Nerve trigger points commonly occur at several other spots as well. Trigger points are deposits of fibrous tissue, also called fibrosis, that accumulate on nerves of the arm, often where the nerves give branches to muscles. They bind or "tether" the nerve in place, and pinch or tug on the nerve when you move. Like the tender spots of the muscle spasms, you will not feel these spots unless someone presses on them. More likely, you will feel what doctors call "referred" pain or numbness in the fingers that the particular nerve innervates. Another theory attributes some of the nerve trauma to the fact that the nerves actually shorten due to the static work position. Whichever cause contributes to your condition, the result is the same: nerve aggravation, and if untreated, damage.

That's it. That's how you arrive at a state where you feel either pain or erratic numbness at inexplicable times, without specific events to which you can attach them. We don't suggest that you will have every one of these aspects of the problem, but the larger picture is very likely to be accurate if you've been typing for several years and start to notice problems. Your entire upper extremity, has been deconditioned by working in a static position, and overwhelmed by constant tension. It reacts with its normal healing mechanisms but they don't have time to do their usual magic.

This brings us to what we call the unfortunate physiological truth of RSI:

#1 Physiological Truth of RSI

For better or worse, the bones and tendons, and to a lesser extent the muscles (collectively the musculoskeletal system) will try to adapt to almost any habitual posture and activity. Unfortunately, they will do this with no accommodation whatsoever to the nervous system, which has no such adaptability. The nerves weave their way through a harsh, super-high-stress labyrinth of muscle and tendons and send back the news, as best they can. As your body struggles to accommodate the monotonous, tiring posture of keyboard work the news itself gets worse over time, and the nerves themselves, in their role as messengers, become so battered they can no longer do their jobs.

The nerves get trapped or traumatized in any number of spots on the way from the brain to the fingertips. Whether you will develop some of these spots, or which spot you will develop first is anyone's guess. You may be lucky and not develop problems. If you are not so lucky, the decision you must make is whether it is appropriate to regard one of these spots as a problem unto itself or as part of the larger scenario that we've described.

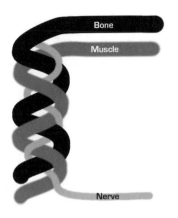

What It's Like to Be a Nerve in a Typist's Arm

Nerves weave their way through a miraculous arrangement of muscle and bone. This design is good enough for a lifetime of use and even frequent abuse, but it's not good enough for 10 years of day-long typing... if you fall victim to any RSI tendencies.

To begin to judge the big picture for yourself, consider just the following piece of information for a moment: many patients report temporary relief from surgery, after which symptoms recur. (Do you recall the story of Case Study A, that we asked you to remember?) This is a striking phenomenon... think about the implications carefully. If the surgery didn't work *at all*, we could easily explain that it failed to address the disease at all. But how could it work only temporarily? The answer is that it addressed the symptoms, not the cause. By relieving pressure at one of the trouble spots, perhaps just at the wrist (the most notorious of all the trouble spots), the trauma to the nerve is greatly reduced. But all liquids, such as the fluids of inflammation, are incompressible. It only takes the body a matter of time to fill the enlarged area again, and you are back where you were before surgery. Typically, the symptoms will appear to move around as you address one problem spot after another.

> "They didn't understand when I said "the pain moves... sometimes it's in my arm, sometimes, it's in my back...."
>
> -- Patient B.

Despite the dire tone you will read in many case stories about the supposedly irreversible "curse" if you cross the line into nerve damage, rarely do we believe the nerve is actually damaged. It is certainly under trauma, but in most cases, eliminating the trauma gives you a chance to recover. In more serious cases, the nerve needs substantial time to heal, perhaps up to a year. Too many people simply never get the right therapy to enable healing. They're still hanging by their ankles.

Will the Real Cause Please Stand Up?

As we've emphasized, without an accurate picture of the entire scenario, it's very easy to focus on a misleading target. This is what accounts for a large proportion of failed surgeries that you will encounter in much of the anecdotal literature. Now that we've laid out our theory, you can see there are many intertwined factors. But which ones are causes and which ones are results? And why does it matter? It matters because the most effective solution will be the one that eliminates the root causes.

The following figure shows our breakdown of the causes and effects.

Schematic of the Root Causes of RSI

It's easy to identify many of the factors involved in RSI, but developing a successful treatment strategy is only possible if your appraisal of root causes is accurate.

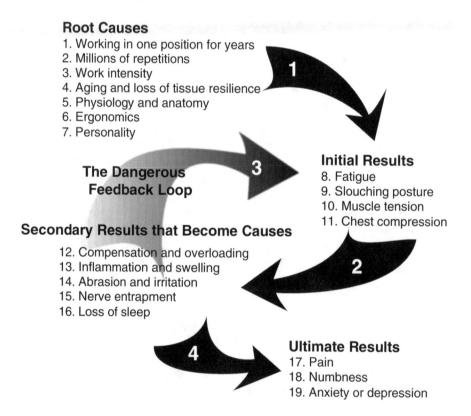

Root Causes
1. Working in one position for years
2. Millions of repetitions
3. Work intensity
4. Aging and loss of tissue resilience
5. Physiology and anatomy
6. Ergonomics
7. Personality

The Dangerous Feedback Loop

Initial Results
8. Fatigue
9. Slouching posture
10. Muscle tension
11. Chest compression

Secondary Results that Become Causes
12. Compensation and overloading
13. Inflammation and swelling
14. Abrasion and irritation
15. Nerve entrapment
16. Loss of sleep

Ultimate Results
17. Pain
18. Numbness
19. Anxiety or depression

The figure shows that, by our analysis, only items one through seven are true root causes. All of the others are results, of one form or another. They do a good job, however, of masquerading as causes once your situation begins to "snowball," as we'll describe next. We can't reverse every one of the root causes, so a fair amount of our recommendations will address the middle ground, factors 6 to 16. Notice that the only genuine results are 17-19—they're the ones that you feel. If we didn't feel symptoms, we wouldn't care about all of this.

The Pain Cycle and Destructive Power of Feedback

The process we've been describing all along is chronic, meaning long-term, not short-term. Your body can recover from a short-term problem by resting and using its normal healing mechanisms. But when exposed to sustained trauma, it is unable to heal. Instead, it starts to compensate to manage the situation as well as possible.

What makes the RSI pain cycle so insidious is a phenomenon that engineers call "feedback." You may recognize this term in the context of a public address or sound system, where feedback causes a loud screeching sound, until someone frantically unplugs a microphone or turns down the volume. Feedback happens when a microphone is near a loudspeaker—a little sound from the speaker goes into the mike and makes more sound, which in turn goes into the mike making even more sound, and so on and so on.

The magic of feedback occurs when a result is no longer just a result, but starts to contribute as a cause, as indicated by arrow number three in the previous figure. In RSI this happens on several levels. Let's consider one such turncoat result, loss of sleep, which switches sides to the cause column. If your RSI symptoms initially occur at night, as they do with many people, they will interrupt your sleep. At this point, loss of sleep is most decidedly a result of your problem. But it causes you to fatigue more easily during the daytime, which in turn might cause you to rest your hands on the edge of the keyboard, reducing blood flow and causing pressure on nerves. Or it might cause your shoulders to drop down and forward, compressing the nerves and blood vessels in your thoracic outlet and brachial plexus. This crossing over, where what had been a result starts to contribute as a cause is the dangerous feedback part.

> "I've played hockey every weekend for 20 years and, away from the computer, am as far from sedentary as can be. But my symptoms developed when I had a project that I couldn't tear myself away from. And it was at the same time my first child was born, reducing my sleep."
>
> -- Patient E

The following diagram takes our cause-and-effect analysis to another level of detail. It helps you visualize how the major elements interact to wreak havoc in your upper body, as the demands of incessant typing exceed your tolerance.

How RSI Attacks You Physiologically

This detailed flowchart shows what you might think of as the enemy's devious battle plan, from the therapist's point of view.

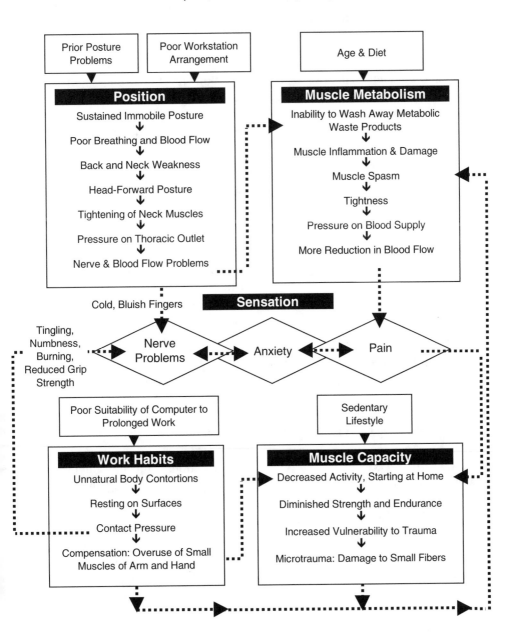

Notice that almost all roads lead through pain and muscle inflammation, creating the chronic cycle that the therapist must break. It's important to emphasize that the cycle shown in the flowchart represents the process once you reach chronic involvement levels and the body can't heal normally because it is overloaded by the cumulative damage and daily assault.

Notice also in the flowchart, in the Muscle Capacity box, that many people start to reduce their workload at home first! Although you might experience the same amount of pain or discomfort at both locations, the response of most workaholic computer users is to persevere at work and try to recuperate at home. Also, at home you are often less distracted, particularly when resting or trying to sleep, so the problems are more noticeable.

Muscular vs. Neurological "Trauma Paths"

Although our scenario explains the general pattern in which we believe the problems occur, we have found that there are two separate paths that the damage can take, which we call *trauma paths*. In the first, muscular inflammation is the predominant symptom, and in the other nerve entrapment is the problem. Often, both will contribute to your symptoms to some extent, because they will affect one another as you develop the classic pain cycle. But one or the other usually becomes the primary focus of therapy.

Nerve problems are predominated by trigger points that cause changes in sensation such as numbness, tingling, pins-and-needles, or even electric shock-like spikes, collectively called "paraesthesias." In such cases, the nerve may be degenerating and you should absolutely be concerned about long-term damage if you continue to work through the pain. In fact, you may be more inclined to persevere because you might not regard it as pain... it might feel like "aggravation" or "irritation." But the same nerves that provide sensation often provide motor function, meaning they move your limbs and fingers. *Problems with sensation must be regarded as early warning signs of potential motor function loss. DO NOT continue to work through numbness, tingling, or similar sensations.*

In contrast, muscle problems are typified by aching or searing pain, loss of grip strength or stamina, or pain when you move. With muscular trauma, your nerves are usually in fine condition—they are simply reporting a very painful state. The greater portion of RSI patients seem to have muscular conditions, and these patients report more significant overall pain than those with nerve problems. They also report substantial emotional consequences since so many aspects of life quickly become painful. Simple tasks like holding objects in the hands, opening a door, and driving a car can become unbearable. The possible "up side" to muscular problems is that muscles are more naturally inclined toward rebuilding than nerves. Nerves heal much more slowly. Muscles are made for adaptability and adjustment. It's only because you've acclimated them to a static, unchanging workload that it will be challenging to work them back into shape.

Prognosis

In our experience, serious RSI problems take about a half a year or longer to heal. The healing process is not the same for chronic RSI as for something like a broken bone because RSI attacks soft tissue and your nervous system. When your nervous system is attacked, your normal defense mechanisms are, frankly, confused and the road back to health will have lots of ups and downs. But don't get discouraged.

When you do get on the road to recovery, keep in mind that your body has declared new rules for the game, and you must forever play by its rules. You won't be able to abuse your body in the same maniacal but surreptitious way. You'll have to learn new ways to work... to be more careful about taking breaks, working in less stressful positions, warming up much like an athlete does before competition, and reducing the overall extent of the repetition involved in your work. But your body has an incredible capacity for healing and your RSI will heal if you address the true root causes and change the way you work.

> What's the hardest part of changing?
>
> "Everything."
>
> -- Patient C.

Explaining the Inexplicable

Because RSI is so controversial and so poorly understood, there are many peculiar aspects to it that are worth special attention. In the following topics, we'll take a more careful look at some of these issues.

It's Not an Isolated, Localized Syndrome

The temptation in traditional diagnosis is to find one of the individual problems described in our scenario, such as tenosynovitis, and fix it by itself. But there's more than enough evidence in the literature and accumulated case histories to demonstrate that most sufferers don't have just one of these problems. The "syndromes" that are alluded to earlier are often presented in the medical community as causes, but in our view they are all results. And you almost always have symptoms from several of them.

This is confirmed by the following diagnosis of one of our case study patients, a very severe RSI patient, by no less than Dr. Pascarelli himself. Take particular note of the "specific" diagnosis.

> "Dr. Pascarelli's examination was very thorough and lasted at least two hours. He reviewed my X-rays, examined my neck, spine, back, shoulders, arms, hands, and fingers and performed tests such as Roos, etc. He also videotaped me typing at a keyboard and then we reviewed the video in slow motion to identify the root cause of my injuries. He provided me with a specific diagnosis including: neuro-vascular thoracic outlet syndrome, RSI/myofascial pain, lateral and medial epicondylitis, postural mis-alignment, and finger, hand, wrist and arm tendinitis. He recommended physical therapy, provided a course of treatment for the therapist, and he spoke with the therapist, Suparna."
>
> -- Patient D.

After being "through the mill" with unsuccessful diagnoses, this patient nonetheless regarded this as a specific diagnosis, because it identified five (or is it eight) conditions which must be addressed. We agree with the diagnosis. Our point, however, is that only a much larger *cause*—as we've detailed in Chapter 4—could explain such a widespread *result*. Contrast the diagnosis from Dr. Pascarelli with that of other doctors who diagnosed this patient with lupus and rheumatoid arthritis! The multiple factors explain why so many RSI patients report that, after employing what had seemed like a successful remedy, their symptoms recur, perhaps slightly altered.

> "I endured various minor discomforts for over a year before investigating surgery. When I talked to two referral patients that my surgeon had treated, they were both encouraging about their surgical success, but both acknowledged less than perfect results because their 'cases were more involved,' so they were still resolving trauma from other parts of their arms. I asked the doctor about this, and he said, quite sensibly (I thought at the time) that his practice, specializing in hand injuries, gets the most difficult cases."
>
> -- Patient E.

In retrospect these stories bear out a far different truth, one in which multiple problem spots are the rule, not the exception:

❏   RSI is a systemic malady of interdependent structures, analogous not to a flat tire but an engine with some wearing parts. The wonderful book, *McMinn's Color Atlas of Anatomy* sums it up beautifully as a "constellation of symptoms."

❑   When one part is compromised, the others are all overtaxed. If you don't attend to the real trouble, expect a chain reaction.

❑   The factors that predispose one part to injury are equally dangerous to all of the parts.

❑   If your symptoms didn't start in the first few years of typing, the likelihood that you have a peculiar, non-work-related cause such as an unfavorable shape to your carpal tunnel, is probably low. We believe that the likelihood that such an anomaly is solely responsible for your problems is so much less likely than the broader scenario we describe, that you shouldn't bet your surgery on it without overwhelming evidence to the contrary.

When *Is* It Really, Truly Carpal Tunnel Syndrome?

We've made a relentless theme of the idea that most sufferers of RSI don't truly have carpal tunnel syndrome. But when in fact, does one have true CTS… how do we define it?

> *Quick answer: You have true carpal tunnel syndrome if the problem can and should be solved by measures applied only at the carpal tunnel area (the wrist).*

Notice we didn't say anything about the causes… whether they too must be restricted to the area of the wrist. That's actually a bit trickier. Let's consider two scenarios to see how they fit our definition: pregnancy and "Olympic rower's wrist."

Pregnancy definitely causes symptoms of carpal tunnel syndrome. I saw it firsthand in my wife when she was pregnant. At night, she would complain of occasional numbness in her hand. This is a well-known phenomenon because of fluid buildup due to pregnancy. (If the numbness is in fact caused by the carpal tunnel, the median nerve would be pinched, and therefore the thumb, and next two fingers would be affected. But she couldn't pinpoint the specific fingers. We'll assume this was the case.) Did she have CTS??? You can see by our criteria above that she doesn't have CTS because the solution has nothing to do with the wrist. In her case, we simply wait until the underlying cause disappears. Let me answer the question by posing another simple question: "Should we slice open her transverse carpal ligament (the ligament at the wrist), to relieve the pressure and eliminate the numbness?" Of course not! Whether you consider the *symptoms* to be those of CTS is a moot point. From a treatment point of view, she most decidedly did not have carpal tunnel syndrome.

Now let's consider the phenomenon of "Olympic rower's wrist." This example is inspired by a fascinating series of articles in a web-accessible newsletter, *The Best of Tech Time*, explaining how rowers were healed of wrist problems at the 1984 Olympics. The rowers had horrible wrist pain after rowing and the symptoms were attributed to tendon inflammation and its effect on the median nerve going through the carpal tunnel. A therapist devised a technique of massaging directly into the carpal tunnel from the flat (palm) side of the wrist. He digs his thumb across the ligaments (on your own wrist you can feel them bump over one another), breaking up the buildup of adhesions. This had a profound, successful effect on their condition!

Did *they* have carpal tunnel syndrome? We say "yes," because the problem was resolved with measures only at the carpal tunnel. But when we ask the same follow-up question as before, "Should we slice open the transverse carpal ligament…" the answer reveals some interesting insights. No surgery was needed… a direct massage technique reportedly worked like a charm. Notice that, unlike computer use, the patients attained their condition in bursts of activity that produced intense motion, not the static, monotonous posture of typing. Notice further, that these "patients" were in a state of world-class aerobic health, so circulation and stamina were not problems. Yes, they had true CTS, but it didn't need surgery. It was caused by direct aggravation of the wrist, and resolved by direct—but non-invasive— treatment at the wrist.

We would also classify as true CTS physical anomalies that result in an unbearably small tunnel, and accidents that cause a broken (or healed) bone to impinge on the tunnel.

Our point in this exercise is not simply semantics, but curing disease! The first step in healing is usually diagnosis. The result of a diagnosis is a word or phrase that all too often becomes an irreversible mantra of the therapy from that point on. Once you are branded with "XYZ complex," you better be prepared to deal with all sorts of recommendations that are customary for treating XYZ, from the harmless to the potentially lethal. From that point on, there may not be much reconsideration of the diagnosis. The label, *carpal tunnel syndrome*, once attached, seems to carry an inherent credibility that goes beyond the weak methods that might have been employed to choose it in the first place. If you allow yourself to fall for this intellectual sleight-of-hand, you may find yourself, like our case study patients, on a healthcare merry-go-round.

If your problems are weakness, fatigue, pinch points, inflammation, and irritation up and down the arm, be very cautious about letting someone perform surgery on what is simply the weakest link in the chain, the carpal tunnel.

References

"The Best of Tech Time," Number 8
http://hoohana.aloha.net/~billpeay/TECHT08.html
Bill Peay, bpeay@aloha.net
The Garden Island Newspaper Kauai, Hawaii

Are all RSI Patients the Same?

We've stated that we will zero in on the chronic, computer-related RSI sufferer, and without laying our hands on you, presume to know what your problem is and what the cure is. Mustn't we be over-generalizing, then? (And we've all been taught that it's not nice to generalize.) Surely one person might have wrist problems and another simply shoulder problems, right? Wrong, not in our judgment... not if you've been typing for several years.

If a given patient has only been typing for a short length of time, say less than two years, then his or her situation may indeed be unique. Doctors would say it is an "acute" injury. The problem might be attributed to a specific action (or event) and by fixing the symptoms and avoiding the event (or action) again, the whole problem goes away. Perhaps you are holding the mouse too tightly, or reaching too far to the keyboard. You stop doing that and, poof... the problem goes away. But if you have been typing for ten years and you have symptoms, the context is much different. Perhaps your prognosis will prove to be identical to that of the two-year-typist, but that is not our experience. More likely, you have exceeded your body's ability to endure an extremely repetitive, long-term set of physical demands.

Consider an analogy to a suspension bridge. Your shoulder and arms are highly analogous to a suspension bridge (actually a cantilever bridge, but this is a book about physiology, not engineering), suspending your hands out over the keyboard for years. If, a few days after a bridge is built, a couple of rivets pop near one end, and there's a crack in the pavement at the other end, you would have to consider one of two explanations: either the parts are defective or the entire bridge design is inadequate, causing unexpected, destructive forces. The rivets might have been forged poorly. The paving might have been poorly mixed. Trusting that the design is adequate, there's little question the situation is "acute." You simply have some rivets that were manufactured poorly, and a section of paving that must be reapplied.

But what if the bridge is 30 years old and this time, in addition to popping rivets, one of the small, vertical cables also starts to fray. You would have to be concerned that the incidents are related... that they have a single cause. Perhaps the stresses on the system, combined with the ravages of time have conspired to weaken the entire suspension system. The foundation might have settled and the main span must now stretch six inches farther than when the bridge was built. That is our basis for generalizing. Most of what are regarded, by conventional diagnostic wisdom, as localized problems such as carpal tunnel syndrome or tenosynovitis are in fact results, not causes.

> "My initial symptoms in 1995 consisted of nagging pain in my right thumb, forearm, and elbow. Over the past three years the symptoms have come and gone in a somewhat repeating fashion, each time gradually moving up my body. Today, my symptoms settle in my thoracic area and all the connected tissues and muscles, the back, neck, shoulders, arms, and hands."
>
> -- Patient B.

Any therapy that attempts to simply "repave the road" is destined to fail. Continuing the analogy, imagine if several engineers of aging bridges were sitting around discussing their popping rivets and cracking asphalt, oblivious to the collapsing superstructures. We would rightfully suspect them of outrageous negligence.

The Seduction of "Double Crush"

Related to the issue of whether your problem is localized or systemic, is a phenomenon that has taken on the dramatic name, "double crush." Double crush refers to the belief that one's problems are caused not by one isolated, acute problem area but by two. For instance, a patient who has had unsuccessful wrist surgery might later be diagnosed with symptoms in the upper arm, chest, or neck. He or she responds more favorably to therapy on this second area, and is sold on the notion that both areas were problems, as if the magic number were two, not one.

However, there are other, more likely explanations for the greater success on the patient's second go-round. One possibility is that the second trouble spot is simply number two out of three, four, or even more trouble spots... resolving any of these spots adds to the relief. This is especially true because the chronic sufferer is desperate to acknowledge any relief—they are an "easy sale."

Another possibility, unfortunately, is that the first remedy had no viability whatsoever, and the second diagnosis was at the hands of a practitioner more knowledgeable in the patterns of computer-related RSI. The first might simply have been an incorrect diagnosis; the second was right.

> "I had injections on my wrists that didn't work. I had surgery on both wrists that didn't work. I was sent to various therapies, including work hardening, which caused me more pain.
>
> "Then I was diagnosed by Suparna with thoracic outlet syndrome, clearly evident [with the right expertise] by the bluish color of my fingertips... but none of my previous doctors picked it up. After years in and out of work, I was gradually back at almost full time work in a matter of months with no drugs, fancy electrical solutions, or surgery."
>
> -- Patient A

The only magic number is one. You have one body... one system for holding your hands out over the keyboard for countless hours... one set of muscles, nerves, and blood vessels, tightly intertwined along your humerus, radius, and ulna in a beautiful design. But it is a design that is intended for motion, not a static position. The design can easily accommodate millions of periodic bursts of tension and movement, but not thousands of incessant nine-to-five shifts... at least not for everyone.

Symptoms at Night

One of the peculiarities of RSI is that some patients notice their first symptoms at night. More accurately, however, it's the nighttime symptoms that are aggravating enough to spur us into action. Typical RSI sufferers might first have minor symptoms such as irritation or aching in the daytime, but have outright pain or numbness at night. Why is this? Answer: in the daytime, you are in more frequent motion.

During the daytime, the swelling that pinches nerves is mitigated by the massage-like action of being in motion when you work or move about. This diverts away the fluid that would otherwise build up in inflamed tissues. At night, with no motion the fluid accumulates. This is actually a "normal," recuperative response of the body to give muscles a chance to heal. Unfortunately, it doesn't help you sleep, as the inflammation aggravates your nerves and wakes you up.

If your situation is primarily nerve related, another scenario can play out at night. If a nerve has been constantly traumatized or pinched, it might be more subject to the simple weight of your body as you sleep. This is comparable to having your foot "fall asleep," when your legs are crossed, perhaps when you're watching television for a while. For nighttime RSI sufferers, it might be the hand falling asleep because one of the nerves in the arm is pressed against the mattress or pinched in an awkward position. A healthier nerve might not be so susceptible to the same amount of pressure.

> "I would frequently wake up at night with my hand numb. It seemed to always occur when sleeping on my stomach, with my arm out over my head, palm down. I've gotten consistent results from using a gel-filled pad around my elbow when I sleep. I've never woken up when I've used it. I think my ulnar nerve where it goes around the "funny bone" is prone to being pressed against the mattress by the weight of my arm, and the pad prevents this."
>
> -- Patient E.

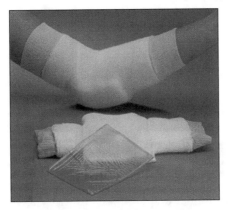

Elbow Pad for Nighttime Use

This simple gel-filled pad may prevent awakening at night because of numbness of the two smallest fingers. But don't mistake it for a remedy for chronic RSI, which we describe throughout the remainder of the book.

Another factor is that in the daytime, you are distracted. Your attention is directed to so many things that the symptoms, *when they are still minor,* are subconsciously suppressed by many of the hundreds of other signals that is bombard your brain.

References

Rolyan® Elbow/Heel Protector with Akton Pad
Smith & Nephew Rehabilitation Products
http://www.easy-living.com/index.html

Predisposing Factors

The following questionnaire spells out our criteria, or warning signs, for susceptibility to chronic RSI. The results won't in any way determine if you have RSI—that's a matter of diagnosis, determined by some direct observations and tests. It can, however, help you judge whether you should regard a single RSI symptom as a danger sign of more serious possibilities down the road, or accept it as a minor injury that might go away with a little rest and prevention.

If you don't currently have any aches and pains, and you're reading simply for understanding and prevention, the results of the questionnaire might give you a good look into your future. If you answer *Definitely* to many of the questions, you might be encouraged to get more serious about prevention.

We've made no attempt to disguise where we stand—notice that some questions have "yes" first; others have "no" first.

Susceptibility Questionairre

Do you hate to walk away from an unsolved problem or incomplete job?	❑ N	❑ Y	❑ Definitely Yes
Do you love your work?	❑ N	❑ Y	❑ Definitely Yes
Do you always look for the most efficient way to use the computer?	❑ N	❑ Y	❑ Definitely Yes
Are you a perfectionist?	❑ N	❑ Y	❑ Definitely Yes
Do you think about work in non-work time?	❑ N	❑ Y	❑ Definitely Yes
Have you been typing as a major portion of your job for more than 5 years?	❑ N	❑ Y	❑ Definitely Yes

Are you obsessive? That is, when you start something do you get "carried away?"	❏ N	❏ Y	❏ Definitely Yes
Are you detail oriented?	❏ N	❏ Y	❏ Definitely Yes
Are you sedentary away from work?	❏ N	❏ Y	❏ Definitely Yes
Do you get as much sleep as you'd like?	❏ Y	❏ N	❏ Definitely No
Are you under a lot of pressure?	❏ N	❏ Y	❏ Definitely Yes
Do you get high-activity exercise more than once a week?	❏ Y	❏ N	❏ Definitely No
Are you over 40 years old?	❏ N	❏ Y	❏ Definitely Yes
Do you use a highly adjustable keyboard tray?	❏ Y	❏ N	❏ Definitely No
Do you use a highly adjustable chair?	❏ Y	❏ N	❏ Definitely No
Do you notice that minor injuries heal more slowly than they used to?	❏ N	❏ Y	❏ Definitely Yes
Do you notice that your joints ache more than they used to when you wake up in the morning… or when you stand up after sitting… or the day after you do strenuous activity?	❏ N	❏ Y	❏ Definitely Yes
Has it been more than a year since you've had your eyesight checked?	❏ N	❏ Y	❏ Definitely Yes

If you've indicated several answers in the "Definitely" column, we'd like to talk to you in our examining room. Step inside, please.

Understanding the Predisposing Factors

The Susceptibility Questionnaire is simply our estimation of common denominators among RSI patients with serious conditions. None of the criteria are intended to be strict or absolute—many folks type for years with no problem, and others make every ergonomic mistake in the book with no penalty. That's life in the big city. But if you've noticed problems, especially numbness, pins-and-needles, or tingling, then your answers to the survey can help you determine how serious you should get about treating your condition. If you answered yes to a fair number of the questions, you'd be wise to regard your situation as a serious, potentially chronic RSI case, rather than an isolated ache or pain. Even if it is an isolated ache or pain, you can't go wrong by being careful. Employ as many or as few of our recommendations as you think are warranted based on how it all adds up, and adjust accordingly as time passes by. Now let's examine some of the individual criteria in the questionnaire.

How Do You Spell Workaholic? Does the following quote sound like it could be you:

> "I hate having nothing to do."
>
> -- RSI Sufferer on the Web

The single, over-riding factor that makes you most likely to get RSI is being a maniacal worker. Contrary to what might be in the minds of some who wonder if RSI sufferers are malingering malcontents who want to take a free ride on "the system," our experience is quite the opposite. Make a list of the top producers at your organization. The RSI victims will probably have a disproportionately high representation among them. These people are serious, detail-oriented perfectionists. They love their work, hate to walk away from an unsolved problem, look for the most efficient way to work (so they can get more work done), and think about work all the time. You get the idea. These folks probably invite pressure and the stress that comes with it because they get the big jobs. It's a fairly well acknowledged rule for managers, that you should give the most important jobs to the busiest people... they're the busiest because they take on the most work. And the cycle builds on itself.

We asked our case study patients, *"Do you believe your work style contributed to your condition? Here are typical responses:*

> "I definitely think my emotional profile contributed to my condition. I truly enjoy coding. I like to do a good job even if that means working long hours. I also tended to get lost in the computer and not take any breaks"
>
> -- Patient A

> "Definitely! Type A all the way especially in the work environment. Good is never good enough. I can just finish this one more thing. I'll just do it myself so I know it gets done right."
>
> -- Patient B

> "Gave 110% of personal time and energy every day for 15 years. Thought they couldn't survive without me. Perfectionist with tasks. Unrealistic self-imposed goals."
>
> -- Patient C

> "Absolutely. I am a very energetic, enthusiastic and passionate person and I am competitive and ambitious. This emotional profile has led me to throw myself into my work, for many years I worked long hours and even on weekends. Not only did I work a lot, but my work really mattered to me. Because it had such importance to me, my stress level was often very high."
>
> -- Patient D

If you could change your behavior to reduce only one of your predisposing factors, you should probably choose this one, your work obsession. This means somehow reducing the tension level with which you attack your work. Much more on that later.

How Long Have You Been Typing? I used to wonder if age was a factor in computer-related RSI, but now that computers are introduced in grade school, it's not age—it's "typing-years" that matter... perhaps combined with age. More young people are indeed showing up at the therapist's doorstep. Combine a fierce work style with years behind the keyboard and you have the core ingredients for RSI. This highlights the possibility that the name *cumulative trauma disorder* may indeed be more accurate. It is the accumulation of tension on the musculoskeletal system that sets the stage.

Our case study patients had been typing for 6, 9, 10, 11, 13, and 14 years when they started developing RSI symptoms.

The Aging Factor The questions about how slowly you heal, and whether you ache after being in one position for a while refer to the general effects of aging. The critical body tissue involved in aging and its relationship to RSI is connective tissue, the material that comprises your tendons, ligaments, and fascia. Fascia is the sinewy material that covers muscles, nerves, and just about everything in the body, for that matter. By some accounts, the body slowly dehydrates as it ages… and the effect of this is most pronounced on connective tissue. If you notice that you're not as flexible or resilient as you once were, it's more likely that you will pay a price for habitual overexertion. We'll discuss more about connective tissue in our discussion of anatomy.

Sedentary Lifestyle This one's an interesting call. I have a relatively serious RSI case, but I'm far from sedentary and the anecdotal literature seems to tell of many active people who have RSI. Maybe if I were less active, I would have developed RSI after 5 years instead of 13. Perhaps our amount of exercise and other physical activity is not enough to counteract the 8-hour daily dose of static computer posture. Certainly, I exercise much less than I type. In any case, the less activity you give your arms, the more of an advantage you give the destructive forces of RSI.

> "I used to be very active, playing volleyball and other sports all the time, but haven't kept up with it lately. I think that's part of the reason my shoulders got so weak."
>
> -- Patient F.

Getting Enough Sleep? Every theorist seems to put sleep (the ultimate sedentary activity?), on the helpful side of the scale. Who are we to disagree? Sleep is restorative. For the first two years of my RSI symptoms, a good night's sleep would alleviate them, seductively resetting my personal doomsday clock so I could go out and tear up my arms again another day. The most important part about sleep is simply that it's eight hours during which you're not typing. But beyond that, your tissues can recuperate and regain some of their normal flexibility and stamina. As far as the early onset of RSI for an individual, stamina is the key. If you get enough sleep, your shoulder muscles have the stamina to keep your upper torso from collapsing into the nerve network that innervates the arms. The "suspension bridge" therefore maintains the configuration in which it was designed to operate. In addition, the small muscle bands that activate the fingers have the stamina to work without inflammation.

There's also some evidence that only an intense level of sleep is restorative. In other words, you must fall *deeply* asleep before sleep yields substantial, recuperative benefits. If your sleep is lacking, the stage is set for RSI. If the shortage of sleep is chronic—as it might be if you are under psychological stress, or if you have young children who often need attention at night—the risk is higher. These are factors that some believe contribute to a higher incidence of RSI in women.

Workstation Ergonomics In our context, ergonomics means working in the healthiest position, which means the most unstressed or "neutral" position. Your neck should be comfortably supporting your head, your spine should be in a natural S-curve, your arms touching the keyboard and mouse without reaching out, wrists unbent, and fingers relaxed.

Ergonomics is in the common-sense-but-unsubstantiated category of RSI explanations. It's conceivable that you might work at the most uncomfortable workstation imaginable, and survive unscathed until your other predisposing factors put you in the danger zone. But the voluminous experience of individuals *once they have RSI* bears out the difference between good ergonomics and bad. I can reproduce a little scenario, on demand, that demonstrates bad ergonomics: I face my phone, put the phone handset between my ear and shoulder, twist only my upper torso from my phone to my keyboard (45 degrees), and type. In a few moments all five fingers of one hand start to get pins-and-needles. Many sufferers can distinguish the difference between straight wrists and bent, some within moments. It only makes sense to assume that these stressful positions are accumulating trauma in the pre-symptomatic typist. We'll describe ergonomics extensively, in our section on therapy.

Other Factors: Disease, Medical History, Anatomy The factors we've listed above are the ones we consider to be the classics for inducing the typical computer-related syndrome. But there are other causes of the various RSI symptoms, and we don't want to entirely discount these. Only an in-depth medical evaluation can determine if your problems stem from causes such as these: genetics, hormone problems, diabetes, broken bones, and anatomical irregularities (for instance, an extra rib pinching the thoracic outlet).

In some cases, the shape or relative sizes of your bones could predispose you to injury by repetitive motion. Conceivably, your carpal tunnel could be small—one study draws a correlation between the shape of one's carpal tunnel and higher incidence of injury.

Other factors implicated in RSI are as diverse as hypothyroidism, use of oral contraceptives, arthritis, and improperly set bones. The same comment applies: if you don't match up strongly against our classic criteria, all the more reason to rule out these factors with an expert in them, a physician.

Understanding the Anatomy

If you could find a doctor or therapist who knew everything there was to know about RSI... if you could keep him or her by your side while you worked... if there were a machine that could expose your sore nerves and inflamed muscles with the clarity and convenience of an X-ray machine in a comic-strip... then you wouldn't need to understand anything about your body. If, if, if. There is some progress being made with an enhanced MRI (magnetic resonance imaging) machine that shows RSI trouble spots, but it is still not a mainstream option.

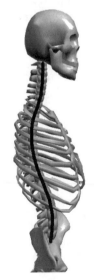

The Normal Curve of the Spine

Until it is, the best option is to educate yourself as well as possible about the structure in which RSI develops, your anatomy. With that in mind, we present the following descriptions of the upper body, from the spine to the fingertips.

The Spine

Your spine is comprised of 32 vertebrae, bones about one inch thick, with cartilage discs between them. The spinal cord runs from the brain down through the middle of the spine, and eventually splits into all of the nerves that reach your hands. The normal shape of the entire spine is a gentle S-curve, but through the course of a hard day sitting in one position, the top of the S loses its natural shape.

As the day wears on, your upper torso becomes less evenly balanced above the bottom of the spine. Also throughout the day, the discs compress. If you've ever noticed having to readjust your car's rear-view mirror in the morning or evening, it's because you're about an inch taller after a good night's sleep. That's how much the discs can expand. The bones of the spine are also surrounded by supporting muscles that can fatigue, contributing to the drooping posture, which starts the RSI chain reaction.

The nerves that operate your arms and legs come out of the spine between the discs. The upper vertebrae through which the nerves to the arms pass are called the cervical (neck) vertebrae. The hands are controlled by three nerves, the median, ulnar, and radial nerves, which we'll get to shortly. Collectively all of the nerves to the extremities are called the peripheral nervous system.

The following aspects of the spine are relevant to RSI treatment:

❑   When correcting posture, you must treat the entire spine as a whole. A change in one part of the curve will result in a change in others as the body attempts to maintain balance. Therefore, symptoms of the neck can spread to the mid-back and low-back areas and vice versa.

❑   Posture problems compress the intervertebral discs and create pressure on the nerves. A well-rounded physical fitness program is probably the best strategy to combat this phenomenon.

❑   The forward collapse of your posture, and resultant muscle imbalance on the shoulder blades pulls heavily on the thoracic area of the spine, the section below the cervical vertebrae. Because so many upper torso muscles are attached there, and it has so little inherent mobility or flexibility, a great deal of stress and compensation occurs in this area. This results in aches and pains in spots that you wouldn't expect to be affected. Not surprisingly, many RSI patients are severely affected here, with symptoms described as tightness or a tingling sensation.

❑   A frequent symptom of patients that have muscular syndromes is a tremendous soreness in spots just under and along the inside border of the shoulder blade, near the vertical centerline of the back.

The Neck

Many RSI sufferers develop their first problems in the neck. In fact, most people who sit at a workstation all day will have muscle spasms, often unnoticed, in their upper back and neck. That's because there are several muscles in this area that move the neck, hold the head up, and support the shoulders. One telltale sign of incorrect neck positioning is that the borders of the collarbone become indistinguishable, because of tight neck and upper chest muscles.

Some aspects of neck anatomy were touched on in our discussion of the spine. Here are some additional considerations specifically regarding the neck:

❏ Neck pain often results in headaches due to the attachment of the muscles at the base of the skull. Some patients report that migraines disappear after neck spasms are relieved.

❏ The forward head position of computer users changes the spinal curve. The normal neck curve must be restored by loosening the tight muscles and restoring vitality and strength to muscles that support the head and upper torso.

The Thoracic Outlet

The thoracic outlet is a spot at the front of your chest, between your neck and shoulder where the nerves and blood vessels pass through the rib cage and muscle layer on their way toward the armpit. The specific position is between the collarbone and first rib, and between two parts (heads) of the anterior scalene muscle. Bear in mind that the precise anatomy varies among individuals, which could certainly answer the question, "Why doesn't everyone get RSI?"

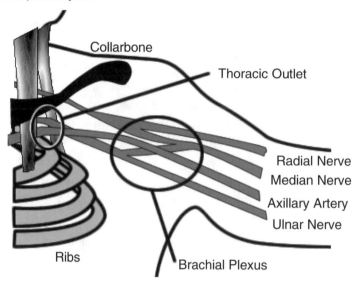

Collarbone

Thoracic Outlet

Radial Nerve

Median Nerve

Axillary Artery

Ulnar Nerve

Ribs

Brachial Plexus

The Thoracic Outlet (and Brachial Plexus)

This passage through the chest wall, between the two heads of the scalene muscle passes below the collarbone and above the first rib. It contains blood vessels and nerves to the hands and often becomes constrained by a slouching posture, resulting in reduced circulation and nerve problems.

This roughly triangular passage is increasingly implicated in computer-related RSI and only recently getting the attention it deserves as a frequent source of trouble. Symptoms from thoracic outlet involvement are caused by compression of the blood vessels, nerves, or both. It can affect almost any spot on the arms, often resulting in telltale blue fingertips or erratic nerve sensations. Many patients also have difficulty holding their hands up in front of them or overhead for a length of time.

❏   There are several non-RSI causes of thoracic outlet syndrome (TOS), including an extra rib, fractured collarbone, over-development of the neck muscles (such as in weight lifters), and posture anomalies. In computer-related RSI, it is caused by the forward head posture, muscle weakness or tightness, and the nature of the job, which eventually cause the scalene muscles to pinch the area.

❏   As many as 60-80% of normal (asymptomatic) individuals test *positive* (!) for some symptoms of thoracic outlet syndrome, so interpreting the evidence requires the judgment of an experienced RSI practitioner.

❑ Several of our patients have been misdiagnosed with carpal tunnel syndrome, when it eventually proved to be a thoracic outlet problem.

❑ In TOS cases, nerve compression seems to be more common than problems with blood circulation, and it is usually the ulnar nerve that is affected, which goes to the pinkie and ring fingers.

❑ With a good examination and symptom history, a practitioner who has kept current on RSI issues should be able to identify whether you have nerve or circulatory involvement at the thoracic outlet. The key is often in how detailed the fact-finding is.

Brachial Plexus

Interestingly, the three nerves to the hand don't come out of the spine one at a time, in three distinct strands. Instead, portions of the spinal cord come out at various vertebrae and are braided together in a somewhat criss-cross fashion, called a plexus. It is here that they form the distinct nerves of the peripheral nervous system. This design probably improves the chances for survival if one of the individual vertebral outlets is damaged. If this were to occur, you might be able to recover more functionality by virtue of the criss-crossing than if each nerve were isolated all the way from fingertip to brain. There are several plexuses (plexi?) in the body. The one that forms the three arm nerves is called the brachial plexus.

Why is this significant to RSI? As you'll learn shortly, the three main nerves that innervate the hand are somewhat neatly allocated among the fingers, as follows. The radial nerve controls the muscles on the back of the wrist and hand. The ulnar nerve controls the pinkie and half of the ring finger. The median nerve controls the rest. So when you have RSI symptoms, the first diagnostic question will be "which fingers are causing you trouble?" But if you have shifting symptoms that don't neatly follow one nerve or the other, the problem might be above the point at which the nerves become three separate strands. The symptoms might be from aggravation at the brachial plexus or even the cervical disks.

Branches of the brachial plexus also supply the neck muscles, shoulder blade muscles, and muscles of the arms. Thus, treating problems at the brachial plexus area can relieve symptoms of the neck, mid-back and arms. We'll be moving continuously down the arm in our discussion, so let's describe the stars of the show at this point, the median and ulnar nerves.

Median Nerve

The median nerve controls the thumb, the two large fingers, and half of the ring finger, but not all individuals are identical. It controls sensation and motion, also called motor control. Starting at the brachial plexus, the nerve goes through the chest wall at the thoracic outlet, then under the pectoral muscles into and through the armpit. It continues along the inside of the upper arm, crosses over the inside of the elbow (when the palm is up), under the big forearm muscles, and through the notorious carpal tunnel to the fingers.

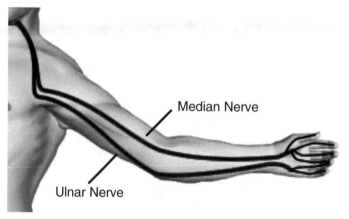

The Paths of the Median and Ulnar Nerves

These two nerves are involved in most RSI problems. The median nerve goes through the carpal tunnel; the ulnar nerve, to the two small fingers does not.

The manner in which the nerve weaves its way through this maze, all-the-while allowing for the arm to rotate as freely as it does, makes it remarkable in retrospect that it doesn't get twisted to a pulp. All of the nerves are built for this sort of abuse by being covered in multiple bundles of slippery connective tissue, and they have blood vessels right down the middle of their multiple strands. But you can imagine that there's little room for chronic misuse. Our view of RSI indicates that the nerve can be traumatized at almost every juncture in its dangerous path.

❏ It can get pinched between the pectoralis minor (chest) muscle and the collarbone.

❏ In the forearm, the median nerve may be compressed in the muscle that turns the palm down, the pronator teres. This muscle is often tight in computer users due to the constant palm down position using the keyboard and mouse.

❏ There's no question that the nerve can be compressed at the wrist in the carpal tunnel, affecting the thumb and two large fingers. The issue though, is determining if the carpal tunnel itself is the root cause.

❏ Because the thumb is essentially "half" of the hand when grasping objects, median nerve problems that involve the thumb can be extremely debilitating.

Ulnar Nerve

The ulnar nerve controls sensation and motion of the pinkie and half of the ring finger. As with the median nerve, there are some variations among individuals. It takes the same path as the median nerve until reaching the back of the arm. Then it goes over the outside of the bend of the elbow, in the familiar groove we know as the "funny bone." In the forearm it weaves its way under the big forearm muscles, and significantly, *does not go through the carpal tunnel*, but is more superficial, closer to the skin.

❏ The ulnar nerve can get trapped at several of the same places as the median nerve, but the funny bone is one of the most likely places to have problems. Because it is so close to the surface, it can frequently get hit, and hurt. If the groove of your funny bone is shallow, some believe that damage here may be more likely. A common surgical solution is called an ulnar nerve transposition. In this operation the nerve is moved from the outside of the bend to the inside, and tucked into a muscle to take up some slack.

❏ In many patients, the nerve gets caught in fibrous tissue that builds up in the triceps area of the upper arm, particularly one spot a little above the inside of the elbow area.

❏ Because the nerve does not go through the carpal tunnel, but is more superficial, you can pinch it when you rest the pad of your hand on the work surface. This is called Guyon's Canal Syndrome, shown in the following figure. You can also have problems from reduced blood supply because the ulnar artery is right there with it.

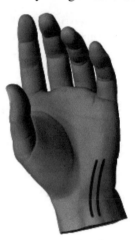

Location of Guyon's Canal

Resting your hand constantly on a work surface can pinch the ulnar nerve and artery in Guyon's Canal, a small passage, just under the skin in the pad of the palm. The canal is formed by a bony projection, the "hook of the hamate bone," which you can feel if you press in this vicinity.

Radial Nerve

The radial nerve starts at the brachial plexus, like the median and ulnar nerves, but then loops behind the arm to give off a branch that controls the triceps muscle. Next it spirals toward the outside of the upper arm, goes around the elbow, and supplies the muscles in the top of the forearm, which tense when you lift your hand upward (away from the palm) by extending the wrist. From there, it runs down the forearm to the hand, controlling the extensor muscles of the hand… those that open your grasp. As far as sensory effects, it is responsible for some superficial sensation in the forearm and a spot at the web of the thumb. Here's how radial nerve symptoms were described, in one patient's own words:

> "… a kind of pulling and warm sensation in the skin, between the thumb, first finger, and wrist. When I use my hands, especially when I type, the spot gets larger and extends into the top of my forearm."
>
> -- Patient from an Internet Newsgroup

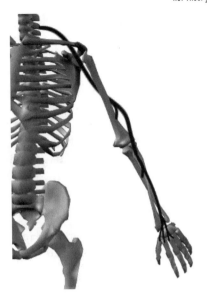

The Path of the Radial Nerve, from the Front

The radial nerve controls the triceps muscle in the back of the arm, and muscles that lift the wrist and fingers.

The radial nerve is not implicated in RSI troubles as much as the median and ulnar nerves, but it does get involved. For instance, the muscle at the top of the forearm, the supinator, is often aggravated if you type with your hands far out in front of you, or if you constantly rest your wrist on the work surface while using the mouse. The radial nerve passes right between two bands of this muscle. If your radial nerve becomes irritated or pinched (entrapped) in the vicinity of this muscle, it can cause an unstable grip, and you can have trouble holding up your hand. If the posterior interosseous nerve, a branch of the radial nerve, is damaged, the main muscles which extend the fingers may be weakened, but you can sometimes compensate by using other muscles between the finger joints. Less likely in computer-related situations, the radial nerve can also be injured in the armpit area, in which case you will have difficulty extending your elbow.

Shoulder

Your shoulder is the superstructure of the arm... its suspension system. The nerves and blood vessels go under rather than through the shoulder so you won't find much in the literature or patient histories that emphasize the shoulder or implicate it as a direct cause of RSI nerve problems. But pain in the shoulder and fatigue of the shoulder muscles are among the most crucial factors in computer-related RSI. After sitting in the same position for ten or 15 years, these muscles are understandably tired. If you constantly sit in a position where your arms are held out forward a little too far, the cantilever stress overwhelms the shoulders and they droop a little. And they roll forward toward the spot where you're suspending your hands.

❑   Shoulder tendinitis is common in situations where constant reaching is performed, so it is associated with the use of the mouse.

❑   Sometimes, if the shoulder blade (scapula) muscles get weak, the shoulder blade "wings," meaning that you can see it jutting out. This is a definite signal that you should have the assistance of a trained therapist.

❑   In other patients, the shoulder blade boundaries are difficult to distinguish, indicating that the muscles on the top of the shoulder and around the shoulder blades are weakened.

> "When Suparna first examined me, it was almost impossible to identify the borders of my shoulder blades. They had rotated from being pulled on by the constant forward posture, and by complete fatigue of the back muscles. They were so locked in place by the muscle imbalance, that she couldn't move them at all, when she tried to restore their mobility."
>
> -- Patient F.

Upper Arm

Your upper arm has two of the most dominant muscles in your body, the biceps and triceps. As you sit at the keyboard, the biceps is in the front and triceps in the back. The biceps is so big that it doesn't seem to get fatigued by keyboarding. More importantly, the nerves and blood vessels to the hands don't go directly through it so it is not a big factor in RSI.

The triceps is another story. It tenses up every time your hand moves forward. And the median and ulnar nerves go right around it on their way to the hand. The radial nerve also has branches that control the triceps muscle. This area is where a lot of trouble comes from. As a rule, wherever a nerve gives a branch to a muscle, RSI problems are associated with the spot. These spots often become trigger points where the nerve is trapped by fibrous tissue. This causes tenderness in the specific spot, but more importantly prevents the nerve from smoothly slipping and sliding as you change positions.

There's one more fascinating thing about the upper arm, namely the force it exerts. Let's work through the math. Your triceps muscle extends your forearm. An excellent example of this is when you do a pushup. If you weigh 150 pounds and do a pushup, your arms are supporting about 2/3 of your weight, 100 pounds, so each arm is lifting 50. Now consider the lever dimensions of the arm. Your lower arm is about a foot long, and the triceps must pull it straight by pulling on the opposite side of the fulcrum, the elbow joint. It is at a mechanical *dis*advantage. Optimistically, there might be one inch on its side of the lever, meaning 12 times 50 pounds of force is applied, 600 pounds! If the cross-section of the triceps, at its thinnest, where the tendons attach, is perhaps a tenth of square inch, the applied tension is 6,000 pounds per square inch.

Now consider what your risk is if the ulnar nerve passes under any of the ligaments that are involved in this huge tensile force. Although it might not go directly between the triceps and bone, on some people it does run between nearby ligaments. True, typing is not the same as doing pushups, but what it lacks in force it makes up in frequency. Closely allied with the scenario of computer users is that of the sewing machine operators we mentioned earlier. All day, every day, they push clothes forward under a needle head, extending their lower arm under significant force. Not surprisingly, they have a history of nerve trouble in the triceps vicinity.

Elbow

The elbow is interesting because it is purported by some theorists to include one of nature's mistakes, a poor design that shouldn't have made it out of Mother Nature's R&D department. We're referring to the funny bone, the groove in the bone that you can accidentally bump against a hard object, causing a shock in your arm. The basis for regarding it as a mistake is that the nerve is subjected to impact, whereas no other nerve seems to be so vulnerable.

If you are diagnosed with reduced nerve conductivity around the elbow, the logic would appear to be that wear-and-tear around the elbow is the cause. Some suggest that the shallowness of your particular groove may be an individual characteristic predisposing you to greater damage. On the contrary, we believe the damage is the result of the nerve being pinched or "tethered" in the upper arm, and failing to glide smoothly through the groove. The poorly designed, shallow groove is however, a likely exacerbating factor.

Another problem associated with the elbow is "tennis elbow." This is an inflammation of the tendons at the elbow. This condition can occur as a result of computer use, specifically from improper use of wrist rests or arm rests, or poor position of the keyboard.

Lower Arm

The lower arm is where most of the muscle-related trauma seems to occur, caused by inflammation. The lower arm has all of the small muscles that flex and extend your fingers. The key word is *small*. Because they are small, they fatigue easily. If you do a simple strength test with a rubber band around your five fingertips, you may find that some of your fingers can hardly contribute to the total outward push. Or hold your three larger fingers and try to bend just your pinkie finger; you might be surprised to find it has almost no independent control. A major factor in the problems of the lower arm is that the whole area is relatively small yet filled with many muscles and nerves. Thus, pressure builds up quickly once you have any inflammation, and the symptoms spread quickly.

Another common problem specifically associated with the lower arm is tenderness on the outside edge of the arm. This is usually a result of typing with excessive ulnar deviation, bending the wrist out in the direction of the little finger. The constant exertion of the muscles that hold the hand bent in that position can create inflammation, starting the pain cycle that then affects the entire arm.

Wrist

The wrist is where most of the suspicion is placed, because of the notoriety of carpal tunnel syndrome. At the wrist, bands of the transverse carpal ligament hold things together, creating along with the bones a small channel or "tunnel" approximately one-half inch in diameter. Through this small opening pass ten structures—eight tendons (to flex the fingers), the muscle that flexes the thumb, and the median nerve. No wonder it is the easy scapegoat for anything resembling hand pain.

It's easy to surmise that repetitive, excessive contortions of the wrist—away from the neutral position—would induce abrasion, and therefore result in swelling. That is almost certainly a factor, but if that were the whole explanation, carpal tunnel surgery would have a wild success rate and folks would run around saying: "Get carpal tunnel surgery and you'll be able to work like a maniac for another ten years." Instead, they say, "I had the surgery, and I'm still in pain." Our explanation is that inflammation of the muscles in the lower arm causes fluid buildup which is most noticeable in the confines of the carpal tunnel. Neither the size of your carpal tunnel, nor abrasion through it is the ultimate cause.

This not to say that true carpal tunnel syndrome doesn't exist. Some people do have true carpal tunnel syndrome as a subset of RSI and can be diagnosed with nerve tests accompanied by manual tests. If true carpal tunnel syndrome is present, and there is significant nerve involvement at the wrist, surgery is a potential solution. However, this in no way fixes problems you might have at your neck, mid-back, and arms... if any of these areas contributed your situation, carpal tunnel surgery is not going to make you well again.

Palm and Pad of the Hand

If you have many other signs of computer-related RSI, you are probably susceptible to pain caused by resting the pad of your hand on a hard surface when you type. The nerves and blood vessels run right under the surface of the skin in the outside pad where the wrist meets the palm. If you've developed this sensitivity, your situation may be severe enough that you can notice pins-and-needles after resting your hand on a hard surface for just a few seconds.

This is one of the few pieces of the entire RSI puzzle that might have a succinct resolution... you stop resting your hand on sharp corners or hard surfaces and the pain goes away. This is because there is no muscle inflammation involved, no fibrous buildup on nerve tissue, and no wear-and-tear abrasion. The only implication of a chronic aspect is that you are resting your wrists because you might be too tired to hold them aloft.

Fingers

In the majority of RSI cases, the fingers do not directly cause problems, no matter how much they might ache. Instead, you might say they are "enablers." They just go about their dirty work, creating this terrible addiction to keyboard use, and messing things up for the rest of the arm. If you feel pain or numbness in your fingers, it is because one of the nerves that is responsible for sensation in the fingers (the median, ulnar, or radial), is being traumatized upstream, somewhere in the arm or torso. As a course of our therapy, we will recommend finger exercises, but most of the actual work is done in the lower arm.

There are some conditions specific to the fingers, however:

❏ Muscles that move the fingers may be affected in a condition called "trigger finger," caused by repetitive flexing of the fingers.

❏ Dupuytren's Contracture is another condition of the hand, in which tough nodules are formed just under the skin of the palm, causing reduced mobility of the joints or muscles of the hand.

The Hidden Structure: Connective Tissue and Fascia

One of the trickier aspects of the anatomy is the tissue that holds everything together, connective tissue. There are three types of connective tissue: ligaments, tendons, and fascia.

❏ Ligaments connect bone to bone.
❏ Tendons connect muscle to bone.
❏ Fascia covers almost everything in the body, including muscles, nerves, joints, and organs.

Fascia is the fibrous coating you might be familiar with from the occasional piece of raw steak that has a glossy sinew around it that you must remove. It creates an extremely tough superstructure out of what would otherwise be a blob of amorphous flab hanging sloppily off of your skeleton.

All connective tissue is mainly collagen, a special molecular structure chosen for its flexibility and resilience. Its unique coiled-strand configuration is very springy. Unlike most tissues in your body, collagen fibers do not replenish themselves throughout your lifetime. Instead the cells of the collagen fibers live a really long time, which sounds good, but isn't. Because they don't constantly divide and renew, they simply get old. Scientist are recently uncovering some of the secrets of aging, and among the findings is that collagen fibers attract glucose, which binds to the collagen springs and reduces their elasticity. If your RSI situation has progressed to a chronic stage, you may have noticed a sensation of wiryness in your arms. That's very likely the effect of your fascia losing its resilience.

Another aspect of the problem is that aging is essentially a continuous process in which your body slowly dehydrates. Collagen is mostly water and as you lose moisture in your body, you lose flexibility and resilience, making your body less tolerant of staying in static positions.

> ### What were your symptoms?
> "Pain and tightness in my fingers, hands, wrists, forearms, elbows, shoulders, neck, and upper back, and at times headaches originating in the neck and back muscles. My pain can usually be characterized as extreme tightness and/or achiness. When I was at my worst, I also lost a lot of functionality in my hands, lost fine motor skills, and lost range of motion in my neck."
> -- Patient D.

An entire army of alternative medicine therapists has hoisted the connective tissue flag. They are called Hellerwork therapists, and their strategy involves treating connective tissue as a system, an organ... something where the whole is greater than the sum of its parts. They rightly point out that the mainstream medical community has completely ignored connective tissue and fascia as an entity worthy of attention. With all of the medical specialties we have today, no one specializes in this area. Without purporting to reduce the entire body of Hellerwork to a sentence, it involves stretches and massage techniques to revitalize the fascia and connective tissue. Elements of Hellerwork will overlap with our strategy.

References

Why We Age, Steven N. Austad, John Wiley & Sons

Classification of RSI Syndromes

This section is like a "Who's Who" of RSI troublemakers. Each topic describes one of the bit players often mentioned in the traditional diagnosis of repetitive strain patients. Keep in mind our point of view, though: most often, the following conditions are *results, not root causes.*

Thoracic Outlet Syndrome

In our description of the anatomy we explained that the thoracic outlet is a small spot in the chest where the nerves and blood vessels to the arms pass through the chest. The head, by falling constantly forward, tightens the scalene muscles, pinching this area for hours at a time. This in turn causes various nerve sensations and decreased blood flow to the arms. The circulation problem is sometimes very evident by a bluish discoloration of the fingertips and may be accompanied by coldness. Symptoms include difficulty holding the hands overhead for more than a few seconds or minutes, and can include all of the general symptoms of RSI, such as pain in the arms and wrist. The therapy that we recommend for this situation includes the following strategies:

- ❏ Centering the head over the middle of the torso, so it is balanced and not tensing the muscles that support it.

- ❏ Manipulation and massage of the collarbone area to loosen the tissues surrounding the outlet area.

- ❏ Mobilization of the collarbone and first two ribs, to increase the space.

- ❏ Stretching exercises that lengthen the scalene muscles.

- ❏ Strengthening exercises for the shoulder blade muscles.

All of these techniques are explained in detail in our discussion of therapy.

Tendinitis

Tendinitis is inflammation of the tendons, due to the irritating, repetitive hammering motion of the fingers as you type. Tendons don't have much if any flexibility or "give" so the incessant action of hitting the keys can cause minute tears. And typing's many forced positions, such as holding the pinkie finger in a raised position can place excessive stress on the tendons. Tendinitis occurs frequently in the shoulder, elbow, and forearm. It is identified by the telltale location of pain, and the nature of the symptoms, more so than any test. For instance, if you have aching pain at the shoulder, elbow, or forearm, and it's not clearly felt in a specific muscle, tendinitis is the top suspect. The tendons that move the fingers are very common sources of aching or soreness in the forearm, so tendinitis here is a frequent diagnosis.

Tenosynovitis—DeQuervain's Disease, Trigger Finger, Ganglion Cysts

Tenosynovitis also affects tendons, but specifically at the point where they wrap around bones in a slippery tubing affair called the synovial sheath. This sheath protects the tendon from abrasion at points such as the wrist by secreting a lubricating fluid. Tenosynovitis is inflammation of the synovial sheath. As with tendinitis, it is diagnosed by the presence of symptoms at well-known locations.

DeQuervain's Disease is pain at the base of the thumb. It is caused by irritation of the synovial sheath where the tendon crosses from the wrist to the pad of the thumb. In this condition, it can be painful to perform twisting motions such as removing the lid from a jar. This condition is often caused by the repetitive action of forcefully hitting the spacebar or an excessively tight grip on the mouse.

Trigger Finger is a problem in which you have a noticeable click as you move your finger. It is caused by a nodule that forms on the tendon in the palm, at the synovial sheath of one of the finger tendons, because of irritation. In this condition, the finger loses control and can flex more-or-less permanently because the nodule becomes lodged under the sheath. It is most common in the two small fingers but can affect all fingers. It affects middle-aged men more than others, perhaps related to long careers at strenuous work. Surgery is often performed to remove the nodule if the fingers are uncontrollably flexed. Hammering the keyboard keys too forcefully is a common cause of trigger finger.

Ganglion Cysts are raised bumps about a half-inch in diameter, usually on the wrist or finger joints, that push the skin up. They are caused by swelling, due to herniation of synovial fluid, that accumulates near the synovial sheath. Ganglion cysts are usually harmless and do not always have to be treated; they can disappear on their own if the source of irritation abates. In the past, they were "treated" rather indelicately, by smacking them abruptly with a book to break them up.

Tunnel Syndromes–Carpal Tunnel, Cubital Tunnel, Guyon's Canal, Radial Tunnel

Tunnel syndromes occur where nerves go through constrained passageways and can become easily aggravated. The carpal tunnel consists of a narrow passage at the bottom of the wrist, between the "carpal" bones and a tough ligament that keeps your wrist together, the transverse carpal ligament. Any inflammation in this area can cause increased fluid buildup... causing pressure in the tunnel... impinging the median nerve... causing various sensation problems for the thumb, index, middle and half of the ring finger.

The Cubital Tunnel is the groove in the elbow (the ulna bone) around which the ulnar nerve glides, *or attempts to*. If the nerve becomes hampered in its usual slip-sliding through this tunnel, it can create excessive wear and tear and compromise nerve function. In this syndrome it's the pinkie and half of the ring finger that experience numbness, tingling, pain, or other unusual sensations.

Guyon's Canal Syndrome also affects the ulnar nerve, so the same fingers are affected, but the point of damage is different. This canal is near the wrist, at the outside, toward the pinkie finger side of the palm. Here, the ulnar nerve and ulnar artery pass between two bones, (the pisform and hamate, if you must know) and some ligaments. Constantly resting your palm on this point can impinge the nerve and blood flow.

Radial Tunnel Syndrome affects the radial nerve where it passes, in the vicinity of the elbow, between the supinator muscle and the elbow. The supinator muscle turns your forearm and palm up, so any twisting action which turns your right hand clockwise can aggravate a situation where radial tunnel syndrome is present. Symptoms from this syndrome generally include pain at the outside of the elbow.

Cervical Radiculopathy

Cervical radiculopathy is irritation of the nerves as they come out of the spine, in the discs between the vertebrae. One cause is believed to be bending the neck to hold the phone against an uplifted shoulder. But it could also be caused by years of static position at the keyboard, or head-forward posture. Depending upon which specific intervertebral disc is affected, you might have symptoms in many different areas of the upper body.

Fibromyalgia Syndrome (FMS)

Fibromyalgia resembles RSI in one dubious respect: it is poorly understood as a diagnosis... so bear with us. By all accounts, it is much easier to describe its symptoms than to conclusively define it. Even the renowned Johns Hopkins has this disconcerting blurb on its web page: *"The diagnosis is usually made after ruling out other medical problems that have similar symptoms."*

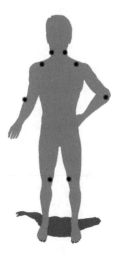 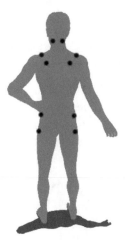

Fibromyalgia Tender Points, Front   **Fibromyalgia Tender Points, Rear**

To be diagnosed with fibromyalgia, a disorder characterized by chronic muscle pain, you must have at least 11 out of these 18 tender points.

Fibromyalgia is chronic muscle pain, attributed by some to improper functioning of a neurological hormone, called a neurotransmitter. The situation is described as analogous to an engine running at too fast an idle. Although there is no substantive test, such as a blood test, that categorically identifies fibromyalgia, it is agreed by the experts on the subject that you have fibromyalgia if you have any 11 out of 18 designated tender points throughout your body. Surprisingly—or is it?—many of these points are the same ones that RSI patients will have.

FMS sufferers are very susceptible to aching muscles when immobile for even short amounts of time. Many FMS patients also have trouble achieving deep sleep. Doctors observe in these patients knots of muscle and taut bands of fibers that form in the muscles. A surprisingly high percentage of the overall population—as high as 5%—is believed to suffer from it, it appears to run in families, and it has been observed in youngsters. Mostly it begins in the 20's or 30's and affects women much more than men. Other symptoms include fatigue, headaches, anxiety, and gastrointestinal disorders.

There is no known cure for it but a search of the Internet will easily turn up plenty of sources selling various dietary supplements purported to be a panacea. If in fact FMS is caused by a neurotransmitter defect, it's not unreasonable that a medicinal "fix" might be appropriate. Only the FMS patient community can make that judgment call. The prevailing wisdom, however, is fairly consistent and conservative, recommending diet and exercise improvements.

Now that we've laid out the fabric of fibromyalgia, what do *we* see? It strongly resembles the symptoms and troubling mysteriousness of RSI. Were it not for the reported child sufferers, pressure points on the lower extremities, and tangential symptoms such as gastrointestinal problems, we might wonder if it isn't simply another way of labeling RSI patients!

We won't resolve this issue in any way, but here's a theory. Presumably there's enough research on FMS that it is known to occur in individuals who are *not* performing repetitive tasks. So there is some basis that it has a physiological or metabolic cause. Perhaps all RSI patients are marginal FMS sufferers, with the same propensity for imperfect regulation of the musculature. RSI sufferers might, for instance, have a slight imperfection in the neurotransmitter that keeps muscles relaxed at the right times. This is not a problem, ordinarily. But if you type for ten years it causes damage that adds up. Perhaps folks who don't get RSI stay within the tolerable range of the neurotransmitter control. It would certainly explain variance among individuals. It's just a thought.

Reflex Sympathetic Dystrophy (RSD)

Reflex sympathetic dystrophy is a condition of hard-to-pinpoint, but sometimes severe pain in the arms or legs, usually reported as diffuse burning. It is attributed to the sympathetic nervous system over-responding to some form of trauma. Some sources suggest that RSD occurs when the body forms new nerve pathways (!) as a response to damage. These new pathways are part of the sympathetic nervous system, which you may be more familiar with as the "fight-or-flight" system, managing your response to sudden stimuli. The trauma that leads to the formation of these pathways can include problems such as injury, infection, tumors, surgery (intended to correct an unrelated problem), and last-but-not-least, musculoskeletal disorders such as RSI! In other words, it is believed that RSD can be the *result* of having a repetitive strain injury. The problem is that these new pathways are a defective overreaction.

RSD is most often found in the hand and shoulder or in the knee and ankle but can be anywhere in the limbs. Evidence suggests that it is more likely to occur after minor injuries, particularly some form of localized tissue damage, than after major injuries. As a muscular dystrophy, it has the potential, if untreated, to cause extreme changes in the body such as muscle atrophy, osteoporosis, glossy skin, and brittle nails.

We want to emphasize that *RSD is a very rare disease.* We present this brief introduction to it, not because it is likely that you will have RSD but because it represents somewhat of an endpoint in the continuum of RSI scenarios. The belief is that it can occur as a result of an untreated, or poorly treated RSI problem. And, like other RSI problems, catching it early is crucial, so knowing what to look for can make all the difference.

References

Reflex Sympathetic Dystrophy Network
http://www.rsdnet.org/

Diagnosing RSI

If RSI were easy to diagnose, there wouldn't be so many people who have had surgery to no avail. If you read the books we've mentioned, you'll see pretty pictures of simple tests and black-and-white declarations of how the tests separate the "haves" from the "have-nots." But you'll read in one case study after another about test results that prove to be misleading after the indicated therapy fails.

> "My doctor ordered an EMG. The results showed that I had bilateral carpal tunnel syndrome. ... I had one surgery in December and the next surgery in February. ... After the surgery, my hands started going numb again within a week of typing."
>
> -- Patient A.

Keep A Log

If you're reading this book because you are starting to experience RSI symptoms, one of the most important things you can do is to keep a log of your experience. An experienced RSI practitioner can make good use of almost every morsel of information. It should look something like the following example, but don't get hung up on formalities... any form of note-keeping is valuable.

Date	What I Did	What I Felt
9/28	Tried lat. pull down exercise at gym 30lbs. Also worked on backyard playset for kids, reaching up overhead with both hands, and tying knots.	More numbness than usual next day. Have I discovered Bellis's Thoracic Outlet Test?
9/29	Working on new deadline	

10/2	I notice my shoulders dropping forward more than usual.	General pins and needles in right hand. Resting pad of hand on mouse wrist rest makes it worse.
10/5	Drove 6 hours on weekend trip.	Burning next 2 days on outside of elbow!
10/22	Started doing corner stretch (across chest) much more. Finally noticed the stretch actually occurring. Started using "kneeling chair" to see if it prevents slouching.	
10/29	Worked for 1 week straight, typing less than usual, but sometimes typing at night.	No pinching or numbness all week!

Sooner or later you'll probably find that a log like this is helpful because there are so many factors contributing to your overall state of health that you can't separate them. If you've got them on paper, you may be able to distinguish patterns that show what your healthy or painful periods are caused by. If you find it hard to get motivated to keep a log, try to imagine this happening to you: you have an extended period of time during which you feel like you're cured... and then you revert back to pain and discomfort. You'll really wish you had some records of all the different variables over that pain-free period.

Nerve Problem Scale

In the course of working with a good therapist, you will frequently describe your symptoms. And you will struggle to come up with just the right words to describe what you're feeling. This section will attempt to provide a dictionary that classifies the spectrum of sensations you might feel, to try to provide some consistency. The first scale describes just nerve problems, the second scale will describe pain levels.

If you have what we've categorized as a nerve trauma path, the nerve is not functioning normally. It is being pinched, pulled, bent, or frayed in some way that either changes what you feel (sensation) or how you control your hands (motor control). The following terms are arranged with the least severe level first. The numbers are an attempt to assign relative strengths from 0 to 100, to the levels to indicate the degree of dysfunction, but they're essentially arbitrary.

0–Clear Sensation This is normal sensation. You don't even know your fingers are there, yet when something touches them, of course, you feel it.

1–Awareness If you're very close to normal nerve health, you may have just a slight sensation like a feeling of tension, or an overworked muscle.

You don't have any type of numbness or reduced sensitivity, but you notice one hand feels different than the other. You probably would never discern this level of sensitivity as you *develop* symptoms—you'll probably ignore it—but you might notice it when you are healing.

2–Coldness This can be a genuine sense of coldness or simply a peculiar sensation from an aggravated nerve. If it is a genuine coldness that is being sensed, it indicates reduction of blood flow and possibly thoracic outlet problems.

3–Hypersensitivity This level is noticeable when you rub or rest your hands on a surface that otherwise wouldn't aggravate a healthy nerve. Velour surfaces might give you the same irritating sensation as if someone is scratching a blackboard, or turning your wrist to an odd position might bring on a distinct sense of irritation.

4–Pins-and-Needles Rather than having less sensation, this level causes more than usual. You have odd feelings as if pins are pricking the surface of your skin, or the sensation of microscopic glass fibers cracking within your skin.

6–Pinching This too is distinctly different from the higher levels because you feel "more" than you usually feel, rather than less. If you've had the other higher levels, your condition is probably improving. This level might feel as if you had tape attached lengthwise to your fingers, causing a tautness or strain.

8–Reduced Sensation This is a superficial version of level 10, numbness. You feel a problem with sensation, but it's not intense or deep… it's on the surface or just noticeable. Your skin feels thick or leathery, less bendable, not supple. You're very aware of the surface of your skin, whereas you usually don't even realize it's there.

10–Numbness This is *like* level 15, *nerve block*, in that you have a significant reduction in sensation, but not as profound or thorough. Unlike level 8, *reduced sensation*, the feeling is through-and-through… the finger feels loss of sensation fairly deeply, not just on the skin.

15–Nerve Block This is similar to what the dentist does to you by giving you Novocaine, or when your leg "falls asleep." The nerve is blocked. You feel nothing other than a thick weightiness. Many RSI patients will get this in one hand or the other when they sleep, and are awakened by it.

25–Reduced Grip Strength This level represents the first stage of reduced motor control. If you've been fortunate enough to have only sensation problems prior to this, you'll realize why the scale is now much higher—when you start to lose control of your hands, pain or numbness seems trivial by comparison.

50–Clumsiness At this level, your reduction in strength becomes not just a matter of degree, but one of capability. Combined with the loss of feedback sensations that would normally enable you to exercise fine control over your hands, you are in a situation where you can't coordinate the motion and extent of your grasp. Losing this level of control of your hands is very traumatic.

75–Incapacitation At this level your loss of motor control is so severe or painful that you won't do tasks unless forced to. It hurts to comb your hair, drive the car, read a book, or open a door. Sadly, many RSI sufferers reach this level, and not always with significant warning time. Often there are plenty of warning signs but many factors prevent the patient from dealing with the problem effectively.

100–Motor Loss This is perhaps a hypothetical level, indicating complete loss of ability to flex or extend the fingers, like paralysis. RSI patients do not generally get to this level because they will stop the destructive causes when they get to level 75. Despite our dogged determination to persevere with our work through pain, the body ultimately wins because it sends us increasingly stronger messages. Eventually the message is strong enough that we are physically incapable of creating more damage. Like the science experiment where you boil water in a paper cup, proving that the last little bit of paper won't disintegrate, your body will refuse to let you grind away every bit of motor control.

Pain Level Scale

The pain level scale applies primarily to individuals with muscular scenarios. In these cases, the nerve is actually working properly. But unfortunately, the message being conveyed by the nerve is bad news… a painful condition has been detected. The values in this scale can help you communicate with your therapist and establish some basis for distinguishing changes in your condition. There are various pain scales used in different contexts. The following scale combines information from several of these scales.

1–No pain.

2–Trivial, discomfort or aching, comparable perhaps to a stiff neck, requiring no medication.

3–Minor annoyance, a mild or dull aching. A moderate bruise might be at this level.

3–Enough discomfort to be distracting, but treatable with over-the-counter drugs. The pain from a moderately serious cut is an example of this level.

4–Moderate pain, comparable to a pulled muscle, but still weak enough that it can be ignored if other tasks distract you. Non-prescription drugs only provide short-term relief.

5–Discomforting pain, on the order of a moderate backache, that can't be ignored for more than an hour. Requires stronger drugs to provide relief.

6–Constantly bothersome pain, but not enough to stop you from day-to-day activities. A mildly sprained wrist would be an example.

7–Distressing pain, such as from a sprained ankle. Day-to-day activities and sleep are difficult. Stronger drugs are not entirely effective.

8–Severe pain, on the order of a serious backache. Day-to-day activities and sleep are reduced. Narcotic pain relievers provide substantial relief.

9–Excruciating pain, such as after significant surgery, a separated joint, or a broken bone. Day-to-day activities and sleep are not possible. Narcotic pain relievers provide only partial relief.

10–Debilitating pain, so bad that hospitalization is required.

The Damany-Bellis RSI Scale

Now that we've given names and numbers to the various components of RSI, we want to propose a simple scale of degrees. It's similar to the terminology used for burns—three degrees, with third degree being the worst. Here's our scale:

	1st Degree RSI	2nd Degree RSI	3rd Degree RSI
Frequency of Symptoms	Occasional	Frequent	Constant
Predictability	Unpredictable.		Predictable, you expect symptoms when you do certain things
Severity	Aching, tightness	Burning, throbbing	Pain
Muscle Health	Normal	Reduced endurance	Reduced strength
Nerve Involvement	Tingling, pins-and-needles, reduced sensation	Numbness	

Bear in mind that all of the lines in this chart should be drawn with a fuzzy gray marker, not a dark black pen. This is especially true with nerve involvement, which can be hard to fit into neat categories. Let's take a closer look at the degrees:

❏ **First-Degree RSI** is characterized by occasional, unpredictable aching. If nerve problems are present, it is rarely so severe as to cause numbness, although some first degree RSI problems can cause numbness in the same way that your foot can fall asleep by resting awkwardly.

❏ **Second-Degree RSI** is distinguished from first degree primarily by being predictable and more frequent. If you know that when you sit down at the computer, you will experience certain symptoms, you are not a mild sufferer. Pain and nerve symptoms are not always more severe than first degree, but it is wise to regard anything more than mild aching as a sign that your condition is not to be treated lightly. At this level, you may notice that you fatigue at work.

❏ **Third-Degree RSI** is constant pain, even if it's only constant when working. In this context, "pain" might instead be numbness. (You might be tempted to ignore numbness or reduced sensation, thinking of it as the antithesis of pain, but it's pain nonetheless.) If nerve problems *are* present, there's still a wide range, however. Frequency and predictability are the main factors. In other words, if you have even minor pins-and-needles constantly while working, you should consider yourself third degree. That's because nerve symptoms, when they are clearly tied to your day-in-day-out work, are crucial to address. Third-degree is also distinguished by loss of strength, usually one of the last symptoms to occur.

Now that we have degrees, what can we do with them? We can categorize the therapeutic approach for each degree. We'll see this in our section on therapy, but here's a quick preview: if you've advanced to second degree, you must take immediate action and substantially change your work habits; if you're third degree you need professional help.

Diagnosing Specific RSI Syndromes

Your doctor's determination of the cause of your symptoms is called the diagnosis. But "repetitive strain injury," the way we've described it as a broad causative complex is not yet accepted as a diagnosis. The traditional approach is to identify one or more of the many localized conditions that present symptoms, such as tendinitis or carpal tunnel syndrome as the diagnosis. Our view is that for computer-related RSI, where the patient has been typing for several years, these are often inadequate diagnoses because addressing the problem at the local site doesn't solve the problem. The problem typically moves as you focus on one spot, or spreads out in all directions, becoming oppressive.

Localized diagnosis ignores the notion that your entire upper extremity is fighting a war to hold your hands up in front of you for 10 or 20 years. An over-simplified diagnosis does the most harm when it results in a mechanical fix—surgery—that does nothing to address the root cause. If your problem has its root cause at, and only at the site where you have surgery, then perhaps you will be fortunate, and surgery will be your solution… good for you. If your problem is from your spine and neck all the way to your fingertips, then surgery where you happen to have your first or most prominent symptoms is ill-fated.

There are, however, two good reasons to understand how the traditional RSI-related syndromes are diagnosed: 1) The short-term steps to heal the problem do require understanding the nature of the damage and addressing the site of the symptoms; 2) You should expect to play an active role in negotiating your situation with doctors, insurers, and your employer. Information is power, and you may need every bit of power you can harness.

Understand and Be Involved It is important that you contribute during your visit to the physician or therapist. Tell them in detail about your symptoms, what makes them occur, what makes them worse or better, and how you are limited in your activities. During the examination, if you feel the onset of symptoms make sure to let them know. And ask about what is happening… what the tests measure, what the findings are, and what the logic is that ties the findings to a course of action. Your involvement and understanding of your treatment plan is of the utmost importance. Unless you understand what is happening to you, you cannot manage it. And if you have a serious RSI situation, you will ultimately be the one managing your recovery.

History To arrive at a diagnosis, a good RSI diagnostician should start by asking you a series of questions about the history of your symptoms—how they started, how they progressed, what actions were taken to deal with them, and what makes them better or worse. If you undergo rehabilitation, your therapist, too, will document the history of your condition, and will perform some tests. The therapist's intention is not to diagnose you, but to establish baseline data against which your progress can be compared.

Hands-On Exam A thorough diagnostician should palpate your soft tissue and joints, probing with the fingers for any tenderness, muscle spasms, or scar tissue. They are going to check the movement and alignment of your joints, including, the neck, collarbone, shoulder, elbow, wrist, and back. A quick assessment of the joints of the legs is not uncommon, and a more detailed one is required in instances of lower extremity or back complaints. A muscle strength evaluation will be performed to identify weak muscle groups and determine muscle endurance. It can also reveal nerve problems that have gotten to the point where motor damage has occurred. Another simple nerve test includes brushing your fingertips with a very fine feather, while you're not looking, to determine loss of sensation.

The Problem with the Tests Perhaps the biggest problem with the traditional tests (which we will be detailing shortly) is that they are instantaneous, or momentary. That is, they are observations of your reaction to a certain situation over a short period of time such as a few seconds or a minute. Some tests measure how you respond to an awkward position or motion, others your response to an electrical device. But they all fail to approximate in any way the scenario in which most RSI sufferers become symptomatic. Specifically, they aren't performed after you've been typing for an hour... and they aren't performed while you are rushing against a deadline.

"After I started therapy with Suparna and noticed how much my shoulders were collapsing into my chest, I realized why the nerve conduction and electromyogram tests probably wouldn't get an accurate picture of my problems. Imagine watching as someone prepares to hook up what resembles a model railroad transformer to your wrist. Your posture will improve dramatically as you sit bolt-upright with anticipation!"

-- Patient E.

Lab Tests

Nerve Conduction Velocity (NCV)   The NCV test is one of the most widely used tests to determine nerve problems. It might be administered by a doctor or a technician who specializes in such tests. The test consists of connecting a small electrical voltage (stronger than a 9-volt battery, but as you could probably imagine, *much* less than house current) across various points on your arm, and measuring how the signal travels. If the signal travels more poorly than in a normal arm, a problem with the nerve is suspected at the measured segment. This test is very seductive in its apparently objective, undeniable presentation of evidence: "The test shows the nerve is damaged at this point... I guess we should operate at that point, right?"

Needle Electromyogram (EMG)   In conjunction with the NCV, you may have another electrical test, a needle EMG. In this test, very small diameter needles, similar to acupuncture needles and so small you can hardly tell they're there, are poked into various points in your hand or arm while the electrical results are read on a meter. This measures electrical activity in your muscles and is another indication of nerve health.

Magnetic Resonance Imaging (MRI)   Less frequently, a physician may have you take an MRI exam, which provides a see-through view of the soft tissue in the body. This test is expensive and has not had any dramatic ability to detect RSI damage, other than traumas such as tendon or muscle tears, and inflammation. However, some recent research at the University of Washington claims that a particular technique (the "short tau inversion recovery process," if you must know) has improved the suitability of MRI to repetitive strain problems.

References

"Ulnar Nerve Entrapment at the Elbow: Correlation of MRI, Clinical, Electrodiagnostic, and Intraoperative Findings" Gavin W. Britz, et. Al., Neurosurgery, Volume 38, No. 3, March 1996

Clinical Tests

The following topics describe some of the common clinical tests performed by physicians and therapists to determine which of the common RSI trouble spots is responsible for your pain.

Phalen's Test This test diagnoses carpal tunnel syndrome, or more specifically, an easily aggravated median nerve at the carpal tunnel. Hold your hands up in front of you. Flex both wrists and put the backs of the hands together. Hold the position for one minute. Tingling in the thumb, index, middle finger, or half of the ring fingers is a positive result, indicating a possible carpal tunnel problem. The theory is that the test position contorts the carpal tunnel, pinching the median nerve to an extent that would not bother a healthy person, but not so for someone whose carpal tunnel is easily aggravated.

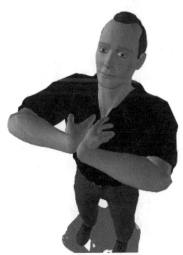

Phalen's Test Position

Tinel's Sign This test checks the condition of a nerve where it may be vulnerable. For example, to test the ulnar nerve at the elbow, tap the nerve *lightly* (!) but abruptly with your fingertip on the outside of the elbow bend, in the groove toward the body. A tingling or shocking sensation in the forearm and the hand is a positive test result, indicating possible damage to the nerve. You may have to try different angles and twist your forearm and hand to find and expose the vulnerable spot.

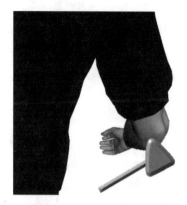

**Tapping the Funny Bone
for Tinel's Sign**

Keep in mind that the nerve at this spot already has a reputation for eliciting a shock, even in healthy people, so the test is very much about matters of degree. If you can find a particular spot where even a gentle but decisive tap consistently elicits a shock, your nerve is probably irritated. This simple tapping test is also used to test other nerves. Tapping on the palm side of the wrist can test for median nerve irritation at the wrist, possibly a carpal tunnel problem.

Thoracic Outlet Syndrome (TOS) Tests   There's no single test that identifies the presence of thoracic outlet syndrome, but a few tests, combined can give a fairly good indication. Most require testing the pulse while you contort your arm and neck. Results of TOS tests range widely from subtle to strong. Severely affected individuals notice coldness in the fingertips, tingling, numbness, or pain within 15 seconds. Patients experiencing the early stages of TOS have more subtle signs such as fatigue, tightness of the neck area, or heaviness in the fingers. It's important to perform these tests over a period of at least three minutes. You don't have to sustain any one of the test positions for three minutes, but you might go through the five tests in succession or repeat them.

Roos Test Extend both arms out to the side at shoulder level, then bend the elbows so your forearms face upward. In this position, clench and unclench the hands. An onset of symptoms such as aching, pain, numbness, coldness in the fingertips, or fatigue indicates a positive test.

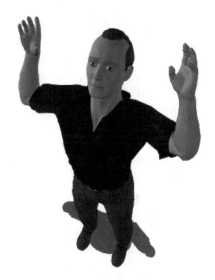

Roos Test Position

Arm & Neck Test/ Halstead Maneuver Measure your pulse before the test. Tilt your head back until it reaches a comfortable stop and turn to look toward the right. Then lift your left arm up and out to your side, parallel to the ground. Rotate your wrist so your thumb turns counterclockwise. Take a deep breath. If the pulse at the base of the thumb diminishes, the test is positive.

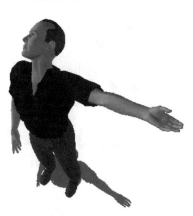

Arm & Neck Test Position

Bent Elbow/Allen's Test   (Not Pictured) Measure your pulse before the test. Hold your arm out to the side at shoulder level. Bend the elbow so your fingertips point forward, and hold it there. Turn your head to look away from the arm. If the pulse at the wrist diminishes, the test is positive.

Overhead Pulse/Adson Test (Not Pictured) Measure your pulse before the test. Lift the arm straight up over your head and hold it there at least one minute. If the pulse at the wrist diminishes, the test is positive.

Clavicle Mobility The collar bone has a precious little bit of mobility that is often reduced or lost entirely in RSI sufferers. You can test this yourself by trying to put the tips of your fingers behind the collar bone from above. If you cannot do so or are very tender in this area, it indicates that the mobility is poor and there is possibility of nerve or blood vessel compression here. Although not strictly classified as thoracic outlet syndrome, because the problem indicated by this test is at a slightly different spot, the symptoms are generally the same as with TOS.

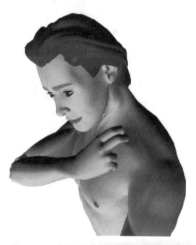

Probing for Clavicle Mobility

For a simple, real-life equivalent of the thoracic outlet tests, try taking a shower curtain off and putting it back on without lowering your arms. If you find it unbearable, you probably have thoracic outlet compression.

Speed's Test Start with the arm hanging down at your side, the elbow straight, and the forearm turned so that the palm faces forward. Lift the arm up from shoulder with the elbow straight. Pain at the shoulder with this action indicates the presence of inflammation.

Drop Arm Test (Not Pictured) Hold your arm straight out to the side, parallel to the ground. Gradually lower the arm. If it drops erratically or uncontrollably, you may have a rotator cuff tear at the shoulder joint.

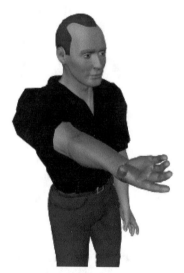

Speed's Test Position

Tennis Elbow Test With your arm at your side, bend your elbow slightly and turn your palm face down. Lift your wrist and fingers upward against resistance. Pain in the elbow indicates a positive result for tennis elbow, which is epicondylitis—irritation of the joint—at the outside of the elbow.

Golfer's Elbow Test (Not pictured) With your arm at your side, bend your elbow slightly and turn your palm *face up*. Bend your wrist upward against resistance. Pain on the inside of the elbow indicates a positive result for epicondylitis of the inside of the elbow, known as Golfer's Elbow.

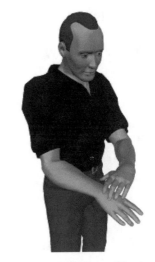

Tennis Elbow Test

Hand Tightness Make a "hook fist" with all your fingers, in which you try to touch the area at the base of your fingers with the top pads of each finger. If you're unable to even get close, you've lost a significant amount of flexibility.

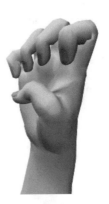

Hand Tightness Test

Pinch Grip Test Try to pinch the tip—not the pad—of the thumb to the tip of the index finger. If tip-to-tip is not possible, and you can only touch pad-to-pad, the test is positive for problems with a branch of the median nerve near the elbow.

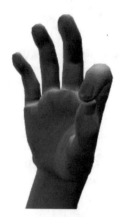

Pinch Grip Test

Finkelstein's Test This test is used to diagnose De Quervain's disease (tenosynovitis at the base of the thumb). Make a fist, with the thumb tucked inside your fingers. Then with your thumb side facing up, move your hand downward in this position. Pain in the wrist or thumb area indicates a positive result.

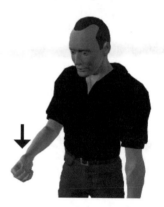

Finkelstein's Test

Part 3: Information

Get Out There and Learn

We've decided that it's important to break with the tradition of putting the references at the back of the book, and put them right here before our recommendations. We have two important reasons for this approach.

First, one of the most important things you can do if you are suffering from repetitive strain is expose yourself to a wide range of information, opinions, and the personal experiences of others. Never has your power to do so been as impressive as it is today, with the Internet. *Failing to do so may be the most traumatic mistake you make in your life.* And that is not an exaggeration, judging by some of the sad stories of people who've missed the chance to treat RSI in its early stages. They've gotten their bodies and egos so badly damaged that it takes years to undo. With the Web's mailing lists, newsletters, ergonomics retailers, medical sites, and dedicated RSI web pages, everything you could possibly learn about RSI is at your fingertips. Yes, the information is raw and unfiltered, but we will help you separate the proverbial "wheat from the chaff."

> "It wasn't until a year after I had surgery, and my symptoms recurred that I started seriously searching the Internet. I was amazed to find how much information was out there to explain pieces of my situation, and how little of it put the pieces together to solve my problem."
>
> --Patient E.

Our second reason is timeliness of information. Some of the information on the web will invariably be more current than what you read here. Are we suggesting that a miracle cure might turn up tomorrow and render our information useless? Not really. A more likely possibility is that better information may arise to fine-tune our methods and maybe even substantiate our position. If a miracle cure for RSI *does* turn up tomorrow, it will be publicized first on the Web... and we'll be the first to applaud it.

Resources

Our intention with the following resources is not to create an exhaustive compendium of all the RSI information or suppliers in the world, but rather to cut through the information jungle for you. Many of the references were chosen because they substantiate our point of view or provide additional detail; some offer access to a wider range of options; others point you to retailers of products we've found helpful.

When you are ready to venture beyond the protective confines of our view of the world, we'll certainly help you with that... the list of Link Pages will put you within two clicks of approximately 1000 RSI-related web pages, articles, and items.

Our Web Page

Our web page has all of the web links you will read about in this section and a synopsis of this book. Point your browser to the following address:

http://www.RSIProgram.com

The Alternative Medicine Yellow Pages

This one-of-a-kind publication—real honest-to-goodness paper, no less—is in a category unto itself. It contains about 200 pages of every non-traditional practitioner and organization under the sun. From acupuncture to zoroastrianism (just kidding), it's got it all. When the individual names are not enough, the organizations might be able to find someone near you. It's available in libraries and bookstores.

http://www.amazon.com or your local library
Future Medicine Publishing Company
Tiburon, CA 94920

Online Newsletter

There are other online newsletters, but we'll keep it simple and recommend one, The RSI Network Newsletter. It's well organized, has a good balance between substance and uncensored flow of information, and there's a fair amount of personal input without banter or commercial influence.

http://www.tifaq.com/rsinet/

Mailing Lists

If you haven't used mailing lists, you'll be amazed at the phenomenon. Mailing lists are tailor-made for a situation such as RSI, which is not perfectly answered by the conventional medical world, and therefore reliant on "anecdotal" information. It's not hard to use one. Just go to the web page and you'll find your way to instructions on subscribing, and then posting messages. It's a good idea to just read the messages for a few days before posting messages.

We do have one caveat about mailing lists. About half of the questions posted to Sorehand will be from newcomers who haven't had a lot of time to get a well-rounded picture of RSI. On the plus side, they are seeking information very early. That's great.

The problem is what we'll call "micro-diagnosis." People will post questions about very specific maladies such as a sore thumb, a particular finger that is numb, or an ache every time they perform a particular motion. And then folks will respond with extremely accurate and well-intended information, in a matter of hours. You will be amazed at the expertise and credentials of the people responding to the posts. But as you will learn from our theory, if you've been typing for several years, all of these micro-maladies are downstream symptoms—trivialities almost—of your broader RSI problem. Read and consider the information carefully. But interpret it through the filter of a total solution to your problem, not just one trouble spot at a time.

Sorehand	http://www.ucsf.edu/sorehand/ This is the granddaddy of the RSI mailing lists, with perhaps thousands of folks around the world reading it every day. Expect about 25-40 messages in your Inbox

every day on every RSI subject under the sun. Post a
message here about the most obscure ailment on the face
of the earth, and five people will e-mail back within 24
hours lamenting the identical problem.

| RSI-UK | http://www.loud-n-clear.com/rsi-uk/
The UK's equivalent of Sorehand. |

Articles: The Great RSI Treasure Hunt

To get you started with some basic information about many of the topics we
address throughout our theory, the following articles are available.

Twenty Clinical Truths About RSI	http://www.tifaq.com/articles/20_rsi_truths.html Bullet items for the "in a hurry" set.
Challenging Conventional Ergonomics Wisdom	http://www.ur-net.com/office-ergo/conventi.htm Credible, informed thinking from an ergonomist. Debunks some simple-minded cliches that are often heard about RSI.
RSI Overview from the USC Medical Advisory Panel On RSI	http://www.ctdrn.org/mhirm/ This is the fact sheet by the moderator of a newsgroup, misc.health.injuries.rsi.moderated. It lists extensive "customers," including Microsoft, NASA, and the US Food & Drug Administration.
RSI Overview from MIT	http://web.mit.edu/is/pubs/is-13/rsi.html Good overview from the no-nonsense, scientific community.
RSI Overview from Two Surgeons	http://biomedical.annualreviews.org/cgi/content/full/8/46/1 *"Repetitive Motion Injuries"* Philip E. Higgs, M.D. and Susan E. Mackinnon, M.D., Department of Surgery, Washington University School of Medicine. Important article in that it strives, as we do to find a common logic behind all of the syndromes.

RSI Overview from an Occupational Medicine Viewpoint	http://www.tifaq.com/articles/occupational_medicine-junjul98-kevin_byrne.html An overview from the point of view of a different discipline.
Olympic Rowers Wrist Problems	http://hoohana.aloha.net/~billpeay/TECHT08.html *"Upper Extremity Repetitive Stress Injuries"* Rich Phaigh Massage Therapy Journal, Spring, 1994 Fascinating multi-part magazine story about massage therapy used directly on wrists of rowers.
Monitor Height	http://www.uq.oz.au/~hmrburge/publications/ijiemonht/ijiemonht.html Scientific study suggesting that the monitor might be better at a low position. But it gets so detailed and arcane that you can also use this article to point out that RSI issues are very difficult to reduce to scientific studies.
Fibromyalgia	http://www.sunflower.org/~cfsdays/fm-rel.htm *"Fibromyalgia: A Guide For Relatives And Companions"* by Devin Starlanyl, M.D. This is a good overview page for fibromyalgia, a generalized muscle pain problem that overlaps with RSI.
Reflex Sympathetic Dystrophy	http://www.rsdnet.org/RSDFactSheet.html Karen Strauss, The Reflex Sympathetic Dystrophy Network. This "Fact Sheet" provides an overview of RSD, a syndrome in which the body apparently reacts to trauma (such as RSI) with troublesome changes in the nervous system.

Searching on Your Own   You won't find specific RSI information efficiently by using a typical search tool. To search efficiently you must use a "meta-search engine." This is a search tool that simultaneously submits your search criteria to several search engines, such as Webcrawler, Lycos, Hotbot and so on. Here are two choices:

Copernic Search Utility	Copernic.com We strongly recommend that you get this freeware (Did you hear that, FREE?), and search with it. You will never go back to a plain search engine again. It provides excellent feedback as it searches, and like all great utilities, loads fast and has a nuisance factor of zero. Where it really shines is the way you see the results… they're all in one powerful list! No more looking through ten at a time on successive web pages.

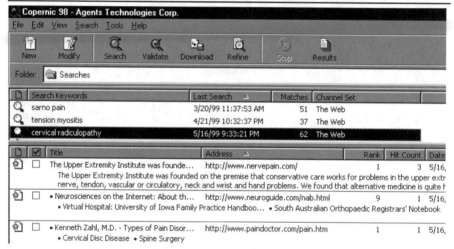

Copernic Results List

This Internet search tool saves your search criteria to modify and refine, lets you see all of the results at once, and sort them too.

Metacrawler	www.metacrawler.com This website is another alternative if you don't want to bother with Copernic. It searches multiple search engines but is not as good with feedback and presentation as Copernic.

Organizations

There are a great many organizations involved directly or indirectly in this field. We'll just show the tip of the iceberg, starting with a good list to explore if you want more.

List of RSI Organizations	http://ctdnews.com/web_links.html Very detailed, but quick-to-scan list of national and international organizations, universities, and research sites.
Bureau of Labor Statistics	http://stats.bls.gov Statistics from the U.S. government to help you understand the enormity of the RSI problem.
OSHA	http://www.osha.gov/ The organization responsible for workplace safety in the U.S.
American Massage Therapy Association	http://www.amtamassage.org/ National organization of specialists in massage therapy.
American Physical Therapy Association	http://www.apta.org/ National, professional organization representing more than 75,000 members.
National Council for Exercise Standards	http://www.exercisestandards.org Source for physical fitness trainers who emphasize strength training to combat RSI problems.

Legal Information

Job Accommodation Network
http://janweb.icdi.wvu.edu/ then click on "Points of Interest."
Phone: 800-526-7234

The Job Accommodation Network (JAN) is a web site and more. The web site is pretty impressive for a quasi-government site, but it apparently has lots of private sector support. Want to know the address of the Workers'

Comp system in your state? Or the name and phone number of the insurance commissioner? This is the place to find it, and about 3000 other, pretty well organized links. JAN is also a confidential, international, toll-free consulting service that provides information about job accommodations and the employability of people with functional limitations. Anyone may call JAN for information. Calls are answered by consultants who understand the functional limitations associated with disabilities and who have access to information about accommodation methods, devices, and strategies.

Link Pages

Link pages provide an anthology or bibliography of the web's riches. In some cases they have a commentary section or essay, and the list of links to other web sites is near the end of the page. If you work your way through the various links, you'll find an entire mosaic of opinions, essays, rants, and dissertations on RSI that you must judge for yourself. We believe if you read a good cross-section of the information you will find that our ideas are fairly well substantiated. You will see consistent mentions that massage therapy and trigger point therapy—two of our primary tenets—have positive results, whereas with all other therapies you will see plusses and minuses. Here's our challenge to you: try to find one article that decisively says massage therapy *didn't* help.

The TIFaq	http://www.tifaq.com/ http://www.tifaq.com/introduction/sitemap.html "TI" stands for typing injury. This is perhaps the premiere web site for RSI information, reasonably well organized and much like a commercial site in its layout. You might want to bookmark the second link, the sitemap as your starting page.
Harvard RSI Page	http://www.eecs.harvard.edu/rsi/ Good general purpose page, covering many topics. Has a student perspective, and you can print it as one page.
MIT RSI Page	http://web.mit.edu/atic/www/rsi/mitrsi.htm Good general purpose page, not as detailed as Harvard, but more structured, meaning separate pages.

University of Texas at Austin	http://www.lib.utexas.edu/Pubs/etf/index.html Stands out for its excellent list of resources including pointing devices, vision care, and software.
RSI-UK Page	http://www.demon.co.uk/rsi/ The European equivalent of the Tifaq page. Nicely organized combination of links and content.
The Dutch RSI Center	http://www.rsi-center.com/ Well organized page with combination of diagnostic info, news, and links.
Oklahoma State	http://www.pp.okstate.edu/ehs/links/ergon.htm Excellent list of articles.
Paul Marxhausen's RSI Page	http://www.engr.unl.edu/ee/eeshop/rsi.html Extremely detailed, sprinkled with medicine, human factors, diagnosis, book lists, doctors, and about 500 links.

Tools, Supplies, Software

There are some excellent devices, ergonomic options, and other work aids that you can investigate but we want to emphasize that these can be a distraction. Your goal is to restore your body as much as possible to its prior tolerance for the rigors of the typing workday. Yes, the conventional keyboard is less than ideal, and the generic mouse design is about as bad as can be for constant use. But don't place so much emphasis on alternative devices that you disregard hands-on rehabilitation.

The following list will give you a few starting points and some of the specific aids—a very select group—that our case study patients have found helpful.

Information about Alternative Keyboards	http://www.tifaq.com/keyboards.html The Tifaq's glorious reference library of every alternative keyboard imaginable, with photos. Also see their articles pertaining to keyboards: http://www.tifaq.com/articles.html#Keyboards

Retailer of Alternative Keyboards	http://www.keyalt.com/kkeybrdp.htm *Keyboard Alternatives & Vision Solutions* http://www.keyalt.com/ This is a web-storefront that offers keyboards on trial periods for a "rental" fee. This is a nice option, because it makes a win-win solution out of the trial problem, rather than just forcing a retailer to honor a costly return policy.
Software Driver for Ad Hoc Keyboard Layout Win 95 or 98	http://solair.eunet.yu/~janko/engdload.htm *Janko's Keyboard Generator* Remaps the keys wherever you want. Free for non-commercial use.
Software Driver for Ad Hoc Keyboard Layout Win 95/98/NT	http://www.kurt.hu/~marczi/keyboard.html *D-System' Keyboard Remapper* Remaps the keys wherever you want. $12 for personal use. Particularly necessary if you have NT.
Break Reminder, with Text Messages	http://www.silversoft.com/reminder/ *The Reminder, by Steve Kellock* This simple program interrupts your work at an interval you specify, offering interesting trivia at each break. Did you know that the infinity sign is called a lemniscate? Or that your nose and ears grow for your entire lifetime? More features are available if you pay the $15 to register.
Break Reminder, with Graphics	http://www.stressaway.com/ *Stress Away Break Reminder* Plays music to announce breaks and displays still graphics of stretches. Free trial, $20 to purchase.
Break Reminder, Animated	http://www.vergo.com/ *Vergo Personal Break Reminder* Free break reminder that shows animated graphics that remind you to stretch and do other activities such as focusing your eyes at a distant spot. More full-featured version is $35.

Downloadable Computer Books	http://www.mcp.com *Macmillan Publishers* Downloadable books to read during breaks, in case you can't bear to simply sit back and rest. Complete titles, in a highly printable format.
The Softest Wrist Rests in the World	http://www.caselogic.com/computer/ergo/index.html *Gel-eez® Wrist Rests /* Case Logic Ergo Products Your goal is to *avoid resting your wrists* on any surface when you type. But you won't change your behavior instantly, so we want you to have the softest rests possible. These are filled with a soft gel, essentially like a water bed, not stiff like Jello. Also found at Best Buy retail stores.
Elbow Pad (for Nighttime Use)	http://www.easy-living.com/index.html *Smith & Nephew Rehabilitation Products* This elbow pad is useful for preventing your ulnar nerve from falling asleep at night and waking you with numbness in the two smallest fingers. The elbow pad is not on the web site, but in the catalog. Look for the "Rolyan(R) elbow/heel protector with Akton pad." It's gel-filled, with four layers of soft cotton, sock-like material holding it. You can probably make a serviceable facsimile by cutting off the toe of three pairs of soft, heavy socks and putting them together.
Alternative Mice	http://www.cirque.com Cirque Cruise Cat and Glidepoint touchpads, alternatives to conventional mice.
Mouse Helper Software	http://www.mousetool.com/index.html *MouseTool Software* A software utility that clicks your mouse when you pause at any spot. You may decide to use it for web browsing, but not word processing. Free 20-day trial, $20 to purchase. Try it, you'll be amazed at the benefit of not having to click.
Dual Mouse Y-Adapter	http://www.cdw.com (and others, about $45) Connects two mice at the same time, to alternate between them, thereby reducing the static position.

| General Ergonomic Products Retailer | http://www.ergosci.com/
Good retail site with leading edge products, such as a break program that even tracks your keyboard activity to determine when to recommend a break. |

Books

General Purpose RSI Book	*Repetitive Strain Injury: A Computer User's Guide* Dr. Emil Pascarelli & Deborah Quilter, 1994, John Wiley & Sons. $15. The book most consistently referenced by RSI sufferers and observers. Encyclopedic coverage of RSI.
Medical Booklet on RSI	*The Natural Treatment of Carpal Tunnel Syndrome: How to Treat 'Computer Wrist' Without Surgery* Ray C. Wunderlich., Jr., M.D. 1993, Keats Publishing. $4. Fascinating 50-page booklet, that may help if you do in fact have a medical situation, other than symptoms caused primarily from repetitive stress.
Yoga	*Recovery Yoga; a Practical Guide for Chronically Ill, Injured, and Postoperative People* Sam Dworkis, 1997 Three Rivers Press. $15. You can ease your way into yoga with this simple book. You may be surprised at how hypnotic and relaxing a simple breathing exercise is.
Eye Therapy	*Improve Your Vision Without Glasses or Contact Lenses: A New Program of Therapeutic Eye Exercises* by Steven M. Beresford, 1996, Fireside. About $8. No-nonsense program for restoring your natural sight. Explains that blaming poor vision on genetics is a sham and the medical community knows it.

Part 4: Therapy

A Summary of Our Treatment Recommendations

Our goal in treatment is to enable you to work free from pain or discomfort. In the most serious RSI cases, a reasonable goal is to achieve a state where you can manage your symptoms. We want to get your body to a point where it is healing more quickly than your work habits are tearing it apart.

In contrast to our approach, you can find several other sources of information that simply recommend eliminating the causes, as in not typing any more. I found particularly amusing the way one book repeatedly referred to "removing the patient from the offending environment," as the best, conservative course of action. That's easy advice from someone who doesn't have to follow it himself!

And keep in mind that simply avoiding typing, although it will heal most RSI cases, is not enough to help everyone. For some serious patients, the routine activities of life are enough to sustain symptoms that only full-time typing could initially bring on. So "removing yourself from the offending environment" is certainly a wonderful course of action if you can do it... we're simply addressing the vast majority of folks out there who can't, or don't want to.

Ultimately, you must manage your RSI recovery yourself. Take an active part in your rehabilitation as you discover what works for you and how your body reacts to different techniques. By the end of the rehabilitation, you should feel confident managing your symptoms as they flare up.

Our treatment recommendations will be rather extensive, so we'd like to synopsize them for you. More details on all of these concepts are presented in the following pages. Believe it or not, we feel that your treatment regimen should include almost all of the following techniques. If you've been typing for years and are noticing symptoms, you shouldn't try to apply just those techniques that seem to apply to the one part of the hand or arm that hurts. That's our premise... you must address the whole arm. The one notable exception concerns the first two items, relieving muscle spasms and resolving nerve trigger points. You might have to emphasize only one of these two techniques.

Deep Massage for Muscle Spasms If you have sore, inflexible muscles, you need to break the hidden muscle spasms with intensive, deep massage, preferably by a trained therapist. The muscle spasms will initially pop under the therapist's touch. As they resolve they will crunch a little, and eventually roll smoothly when pressed. This can take as long as eight weeks to resolve, and more weeks to rebuild healthy tissue. You may find that ice packs relieve the discomfort from the process itself.

Localized Massage to Eliminate Trigger Points Eliminate trigger points that are entrapping nerves with vigorous, localized massage. In normal activity, you won't even notice these spots, but when pressed, they will feel just like a splinter does—a small but intense irritation. Although a therapist will probably be most effective treating these, you may be able to treat them yourself by pinching the spot, and while holding it, performing the movement that the nearby muscle would ordinarily cause.

> "It took Suparna 21 sessions (two a week, 45 minutes each) to zero-in on and break through the fibrous tissue on my ulnar nerve at the elbow. The surgeon who operated on my arm never once probed to look for this spot. When the fibrous buildups were completely broken through, it took another four months to reach a point where my work tolerance consistently improved. The most likely explanation for this is that the nerve took that long to heal. I probably caused this lengthy recovery time by working for several months without treating my symptoms."
>
> -- Patient E.

Reduce Your Short-Term Workload For the short-term, reduce your workload as much as necessary to facilitate the healing process. Take whatever measures you have to. If you damage your nerves, the healing process will take a lot longer.

Improve Your Seated Posture For the long-term, adjust your workstation, your energy level, and your concentration, to maintain a posture in which your shoulders and head are not collapsing into your chest. The goal is relaxed balance. When your head is balanced over your shoulders, the muscles are less tense. Emphasize diaphragmatic (abdominal) breathing to further reduce the pressure on your chest.

Stretching and Mobilization Have a therapist perform active stretching and mobilization to increase mobility where the nerves are most likely to be pinched or compressed, such as the brachial plexus and the area under the collarbone. Restore flexibility, resilience, and range of motion with self-stretching exercises. Continue stretching exercises for the rest of your keyboarding career.

Strengthening and Endurance Exercises Increase muscle vitality and stamina with strengthening exercises. Especially emphasize muscles that hold your shoulders back, hold your arms up, and extend (open) your fingers. These are all likely to be in a state of constant fatigue.

Perform Exercises Called "Glides" To counteract nerve entrapment, perform motion exercises called glides. In a glide, you move your hand or arm from one position to another, without any force or resistance, to put a nerve or tendon through its maximum range of motion.

Improve Ergonomics Establish workstation ergonomics that enable you to work in the most neutral (least stressful) positions.

Use Large Muscle Movements When Working Adopt keyboarding techniques that emphasize the use of large muscles, such as the shoulders and upper arms instead of small muscles such as those that drive the fingers. In extreme cases, you may have to resort to typing with three fingers, or even one finger on each hand. Use the same principles with the mouse, avoiding finger and wrist movements and pinching actions.

Reduce the Repetitiveness Exploit every possible opportunity to reduce or displace the incessant, repetitive tasks of keyboarding. This includes everything from breaks to voice recognition software.

Reduce Stress and Combat Aging Address lifestyle and work habits to reduce your level of work-obsessed tension, and create a more favorable balance between the destructive and restorative forces acting on your body. Work on improving your sleep patterns. Drink lots of water.

Warm Up Do a serious warm-up routine before each work session. One way is to use a hand cream and rub your hands vigorously until your hands get very warm. Try to warm up several times a day.

Therapy by Degree

In our discussion of diagnosis, we proposed three degrees of RSI, and promised to use this as a basis for categorizing our therapy. Here's how our treatment breaks down per degree:

	1st Degree RSI	2nd Degree RSI	3rd Degree RSI
Summary of Symptoms	Occasional, unpredictable aching or sensation problems	Frequent, predictable burning or throbbing	Constant pain or numbness
Treatment Synopsis	Increase strength Increase flexibility Work in neutral positions Balanced posture Breaks	Add these: Reduce stress Massage Glides Large muscle movements Warm up	Potentially all of our treatment measures, applied with the guidance and assistance of an experienced RSI therapist

As you know by now, we don't suggest that RSI lends itself to any iron-clad rules about choice of treatment solutions. But we've targeted two main points with this chart: first, if your problems are occasional and minor, start strengthening and establishing good ergonomic habits; second, if your pain is constant, get serious help now.

Debatable Therapies

Before diving into our treatment recommendations, let's discuss some of the most popular therapies you'll encounter, and see how they stack up against our explanation for RSI.

Wrist Braces and Other Crutches

Physicians will routinely prescribe wrist braces for RSI sufferers who first complain of symptoms anywhere near the wrist. This is common, first because it's easy and conservative. Second, the publicity—can we call it notoriety?—given to carpal tunnel syndrome convinces many practitioners that the problem is in the wrist. We believe that the prevalence of failed carpal tunnel surgery attests to the fact that the wrist is the result, not the cause.

> "He prescribed a wrist brace and said to make a follow-up appointment in six weeks. When I went back, he prescribed a wrist brace on the other hand. He prescribed Relafen, an anti-inflammatory, and said to make a follow-up appointment in six more weeks... if I was still in pain, he would order an EMG test. The Relafen did not help."
>
> -- Patient A.

Wrist braces are a type of crutch, an assist for a limb or joint that is believed to be in need of help. Doctors prescribe wrist braces in the belief that bending the wrist is the cause of all the problems, thinking that ulnar deviation is causing most of the aggravation in the carpal tunnel. Another line of reasoning is that if you have symptoms at night, it's hoped that the brace will prevent the wrist from bending too much while you sleep.

On the first count, bending the wrist outward while typing, the concern is certainly valid... but the remedy is shortsighted. Instead we believe that you must train yourself to work as much as possible in the preferred neutral position. We'll get into more of that later. The second concern, that bending the wrist at night might be a serious component of the problem, is probably a distraction. If you've got all the signs of computer-related RSI, long-term nighttime solutions will most likely be derived from daytime corrections. However, there's little or no cost or risk to using the wrist brace at night, so we don't flatly object to this practice. But we do have a concern: if you match up strongly against our predisposing factors, and using a wrist brace at night removes your symptoms, you may be convinced you have solved your problem. If in fact, you *have* solved your problem, good for you. We're delighted one more person has defeated RSI. But if you've simply placated a symptom, you've missed valuable time that could have been spent addressing the underlying causes. For some patients, this lost time is vital.

The more important problem with prescribing wrist braces for use at work is that it will contribute to the conditions that have caused (!) your problems, namely loss of muscle strength and stamina.

Surgery

Options for carpal tunnel surgery are broadening rapidly, but the typical surgery consists of cutting the ligament that constrains the tunnel. You may ask, "How can we simply cut the ligament... don't we need it? Won't the wrist come apart?" No, surgeons would have you believe that we don't really need the ligament because we don't walk on our wrists like our four-footed friends... so we can get by with less support at the wrist. Others are of a different opinion, citing instances where the carpal bones drift out of position and the hand actually becomes deformed.

We are not going to throw statistics at you, trying to convince you that carpal tunnel surgery has a good or poor record. Statistics like this have always been manipulated to the liking of the presenter. We'll trust that your presence here is sufficient testimony that you have some doubts about the surgery. Here's one experience that we believe is all too common:

> "The doctor said my only option was surgery. I went to another hand doctor to get a second opinion. She said that I could try six months of therapy, which could not be guaranteed to help, or surgery. She said that in three months I would be good as new. Normal recovery from carpal tunnel release surgery is six weeks. I would need two separate operations, one for each hand. I opted for the surgery because I did not want to be out of commission for six more months.
>
> "I had one surgery in December and the next surgery in February. The numbness and tingling went away immediately after surgery. I went to rehabilitation and therapy for each hand. I was taught nerve glides and various stretches. I did certain strengthening exercises with putty and weights. I was massaged, but only at the wrist and hands, especially the scars on my palms. Eventually, they started me typing at therapy. My hands started going numb again within a week of typing. I still had the neck and shoulder pain that I just thought of as normal at this point. My hands would go numb whenever I lifted my arms up to my shoulders."
>
> -- Patient A.

This is the patient that was subsequently diagnosed by Suparna with thoracic outlet syndrome. After a few months of non-invasive therapy, she is now back at work... not 100% symptom free, but very close, and getting closer every day.

Surgeons probably can suggest an operation for every part of the anatomy that might be subject to symptoms. The problem, however, is that in the case of computer-related RSI, the surgery usually treats the symptoms, not the source. They can operate on your wrists if that's where the pain is, or maybe a particular nerve if it's being aggravated at a spot, but with RSI, the pain is often "referred," meaning that the nerve is sending a misleading message to the brain. For instance, if the nerve that controls the fingers is pinched at a point in the chest, it might cause the nerve to send a signal to the brain resembling pain in the fingers. Or the blood supply within the nerve itself might be constricted by the pinch point, causing erroneous sensation further along on the nerve.

When do we think surgery might be justified for nerve problems? When the nerve is so frayed or pinched that the only way it has a chance to heal is to physically alter the structural circumstances that are aggravating it. Some surgeries do this by moving the nerve... some by moving or reducing the surrounding tissues. How do you know if you've crossed this line and it's the right thing to do? The answer has two parts:

- ❑ Part 1: Ask your surgeon or doctor for references from at least three patients who've had the operation *at least one year ago and have returned to the same level of activity you intend to!* If they've had the operation recently, they haven't truly tested their recovery. And get at least one opinion from another specialist.

- ❑ Part 2: You simply don't know when you've crossed the "damage line." It's very hard to tell. Nerve tests are notoriously misleading— many people will test low simply because of their age. Here's a guideline for you to consider: if your nerve has any totally healthy periods, if you resolve well (notice no symptoms) after a vacation, and if you have no motor (strength or coordination) problems, it may be too early to consider surgery. Get a serious physical therapist and get busy applying our ideas.

References

"Repetitive Motion Injuries"
Philip E. Higgs, M.D. and Susan E. Mackinnon, M.D.
Washington University School of Medicine
http://biomedical.annualreviews.org/cgi/content/full/8/46/1
This article from two surgeons makes a strong case for non-surgical strategies.

Palliatives and Pain Killers

We're in favor of anything like aspirin that can reduce your pain. But if it's used interminably as a substitute for eliminating the causes of trauma, it doesn't take sophisticated medical knowledge to predict that debilitation will follow somewhere down the road, while you're preoccupied with suppressing the pain.

Doctors frequently prescribe anti-inflammatory drugs call NSAIDs (non-steroidal anti-inflammatories) to combat initial RSI symptoms, particularly wrist symptoms. NSAIDs will cause extreme irritation to your stomach, especially if it's not made crystal clear to you that you must consume considerable quantities of food and fluid along with them. But even if they directly combat the muscle inflammation that is causing your symptoms, this still does not address the source of the abuse that is causing the inflammation. An RSI sufferer's muscles are inflamed because of a habit of activity that will very likely continue *even while taking the medicine*. The drugs don't stand a chance, and neither do you. The only good bet is that your stomach, which was initially healthy, will also start to hurt.

When might drugs be a viable option? When you clearly have a short-term situation... when your work or life circumstances are different than usual and you don't match up well against our predisposing factors.

Vitamins

Vitamin B6 is reported to have healing powers for nerve problems, but there is hardly unanimous proof of its value. There's no substantive body of research compelling enough for us to recommend that you resort to B6 megadoses. Moreover, there *are* substantial, though controversial reports suggesting that large doses are risky. When we weigh these two factors against the larger logic of how we believe chronic, computer-related RSI is caused, vitamin therapy is not likely to be a solution, and we have little basis for recommending it.

> "I tried Vitamin B6, beta carotene, Proanthenols, and chondroitin sulfate/glucosamine sulfate. Beta carotene and Proanthenols (a proprietary name for one brand made from grape and peanut bark extracts) are anti-oxidants, purported to have generalized healing powers because they kill off dangerous free radical molecules. CS/GS is supposed to help joint health, and is suggested for arthritis sufferers.
>
> "None had a noticeable effect for me."
>
> -- Patient E.

Are vitamins worth trying, considering how easy they are? That's up to you. If your doctor says that large doses of certain supplements won't hurt you, only you can decide.

Cortisone Shots and Iontopheresis

Cortisone is used to treat RSI by injecting it directly into muscles to reduce spasms. Iontopheresis uses electrical signals to infuse the medicine into your tissues without the need for an injection. The medicine can be cortisone with or without Lidocaine, a local anesthetic. Iontopheresis can also be used with other chemicals in localized areas to relieve pain, inflammation, or muscle spasm. Its effects are specific to that area and temporary, but useful until the causes of the damage are controlled.

While there are patients who experience improvement with these techniques, and cortisone is occasionally used in conjunction with the course of therapy that we recommend, it is nonetheless a symptomatic measure. Consider these techniques with the guidance of medical professionals, but use the information we provide to determine if you are unwisely expecting it to be a "quick fix" to a problem that was years in the making.

The Recovery Roller Coaster

Our patients with serious computer-related RSI have taken about a half a year to "heal." Healing is not the same for chronic RSI as for a broken bone. Your body has declared new rules for the game, and you must forever play by its rules. But the good news is you can still do the work you love.

RSI recovery will occur if you have the right treatment, but it is not smooth. There is a very consistent pattern observed in our history of cases, indicating three more-or-less distinct phases, of roughly eight weeks each:

❑ Weeks 1-8: Initial response to treatment

❑ Weeks 9-16: Improvements and setbacks (ups and downs)

❑ Weeks 17-24: Consistent, slow improvement

We've assigned specific numbers of weeks simply to give you some guidance… this is an extremely variable situation. Although your situation may shift these ranges considerably, we have found the 24-week time period to be about average, but your recovery may continue for up to two years, especially muscle endurance. Now let's look at each of these phases in more detail.

Recovery Phase 1: The Initial Response to Treatment

In the initial weeks of our treatment, consisting of massage therapy, myofascial release, and muscle and joint reconditioning, you will feel bruised. Whether your situation is primarily muscular or nerve-related, the therapy will consist first and foremost of deep massage to release bound tissues and break up the knots. This will make you aware of the spasms that until now probably have been unnoticeable. Depending on the number and depth of your spasms, you may feel bruised for days or weeks, but the discomfort will quickly give way to an anticipated sense of relief, like a deep stretch when you wake up.

> "I was pretty sore for the first few sessions, probably because I wasn't even aware of most of the tender spots I had, and I had just gotten accustomed to working with minor aches. I thought my only problem was my hand but it was clear I had problems on my whole arm, and especially the neck."
>
> -- Patient F.

Stretching is also a significant part of the initial therapy, and this will usually make you feel pretty good. If you've gotten to the point where your arms felt wiry, the stretching and range of motion improvement may have very noticeable effects on you. You may notice more "kinesthetic" sense, being more aware of your limbs, actually feeling the presence of your body again. Between the deep massage and flexibility changes, you would not be the first patient to remark that the massage therapy is addicting.

After a handful of treatments, despite profound new sensations and changes, you may not necessarily have any impressive reduction in your symptoms. If it took you ten years to cause this problem, ten sessions will not "cure" you. What you can expect during the initial phase, however, is to get temporary abatement of certain symptoms, as the therapist zeroes-in on your bad habits and trouble spots. Each session might make a little progress, and you may increase your work tolerance a little more. Or it may become easier and quicker for a therapist (or your own exercises) to return you to a comfortable state, as the problem spots are identified and resolved a little more with time.

Recovery Phase 2: Ups and Downs

After your therapy has established some track record of success in improving your symptoms, you'll enter the second phase of your response to the treatment. In this phase you'll notice distinct peaks and valleys in your reaction to the treatment where sometimes you'll feel fine, and at other times your symptoms may be just as bad as they were before. This is especially frustrating because you're so tempted by the episodes of improvement.

RSI responds to treatment in this manner because it's not as simple as a broken bone or lesion that consistently regrows tissue with each passing day, while you're careful to keep it out of harm's way. Nor is it is like an infection, where a foreign agent is identified and eradicated. Instead, it's a complex response by your body to a situation in which the musculo-skeletal system overloaded. When the situation is bad enough, even the nervous system, which is responsible for reporting and regulating body functions fails. This interference with the regulatory role of the nervous system is what causes the erratic healing process.

For instance, let's examine what happened to one patient when trigger points, accumulations of fibrous tissue, started to resolve in his upper arm. The first spot resolved after about 16 sessions and he felt good as new, almost like throwing a light switch after one particular session. Then slowly, over the next few weeks, the exact same symptoms occurred! How could this be? Although we can't know for sure, one possible explanation is that there were multiple trigger points all along. And in fact, Suparna did find another fibrous mass two inches farther up the nerve. Here's how the situation probably played out. The first trigger point, shown in the following diagram, was pinching the nerve just above the elbow. This was causing excessive tension on the nerve from that point down to the end of the fingers.

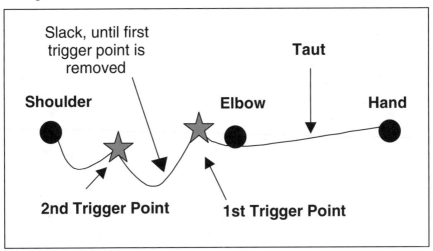

The part of the nerve from this trigger point up to the shoulder was slack. Imagine a rubber band connecting two points. You pinch it in the middle and pull toward the left. The right side is then taut and the left side is slack. If, with your other hand, you create another pinch point in the slack part, you may be able to imagine how it would behave... when the first pinch point is released, the second one comes into play.

This is what we believe happens as trigger points are resolved. Your nerves, with their aging connective tissue, are like the rubber bands in our explanation. In youth, the nerves have tremendous resilience that might get you through several years with some of these pinch points, but eventually the entrapment will create too much wear and tear. When one pinch point is released, you'll have enough slack in the rubber bands that you'll feel relieved for some period of time... until the slack is taken up and the next pinch point tugs on the nerve.

Recovery Phase 3: Slow, Consistent Improvement

In the third phase of your recovery, you'll notice consistent but slow improvement. During this phase, you might notice that you can work for increasingly longer periods of time before the onset of symptoms. You should also notice that the severity of symptoms decreases over time. Some of the indicators of your recovery may not be related to your 9-to-5 work. For instance, you might notice less discomfort when driving or performing household chores.

> "I went to see Suparna three times a week and finally became convinced that I would get better. She worked her magic and eventually I started back to work 2 hours a day. I did this for two weeks and then bumped up to four hours a day. After two weeks, I bumped up again to 6 hours a day. I have since bumped up to seven hours a day and have very little symptoms to report. I am back to lifting weights and building up my endurance."
>
> -- Patient A.

During this time you'll learn what your body's new capacity is for repetitive work. You'll also start cheating on many of the techniques that helped get you to this point in your recovery, reducing your breaks and stretching exercises, and not concentrating on good ergonomics. Your challenge will be to sustain the good habits that helped in your recovery.

How Much Recovery Can You Expect?

If your situation was serious at outset, "complete recovery" means being able to work again with a manageable reaction to repetitive work. In other words, you won't be able to abuse your body in the same reckless but insidious way. You'll have to learn new ways to work: to be more careful about taking breaks, working in less stressful positions, warming up much like an athlete does before competition, and reducing the overall extent of the repetition involved in your work. But your body has an incredible capacity for healing and your RSI will heal if you address the true root causes. In fact, we prefer to talk in terms of "healing" from RSI, not being cured. Now let's see exactly how that's done.

> "Suparna's treatment is absolutely helping me immeasurably. Her treatment has enabled me to regain many functions, and to return to work full-time."
>
> -- Patient D.

Strategies for Hands-On Therapy

In this chapter, we will discuss the many interdependent aspects of RSI from a therapeutic perspective, and describe the specific steps needed to resolve them. Some areas will require assistance from a therapist, but we'll provide as much guidance as we can to give you the tools to heal yourself if a therapist is not available. As mentioned earlier, your therapy should consist of almost all of the measures you will read about in the following pages, to a greater or lesser extent. The goal is to revitalize your upper extremity. The only "optional" elements are the therapies for muscle spasms and nerve trigger points, since most patients have one or the other.

Muscle Spasms

Muscle spasms are knots of muscle in a state of continuous tension and should not be confused with cramps. With a cramp, a muscle suddenly, quite agonizingly contracts. Spasms can be the body's reaction to almost any form of pain, among them the various RSI stresses and strains. When the cause is from a specific point of aggravation, the spasm usually starts in the affected area but it can spread to other areas. This can happen because of the body's compensating mechanisms, and from the stress of the symptoms and your reaction to it. You generally do not feel the spasm itself, unlike a pulled muscle, or an acute spasm associated with an event, because these spasms are chronic.

The Normal Healing Process When the body experiences a trauma such as small tears in muscle fibers from prolonged activity, it responds with a muscle spasm. The spasm is accompanied by an inflammatory response to try to heal the damage. The inflammation leads to the formation of metabolites in the area. In a normal, healthy recovery scenario, the metabolites are eventually washed away by the blood flow, resulting in healing and reduced spasm.

Which Muscles Are Affected? In general terms, the muscles affected by prolonged computer use include those of the entire arm and hand, neck, mid-back and occasionally the low back. The common areas of muscle spasm noted in a patient with RSI are shown in the following diagrams:

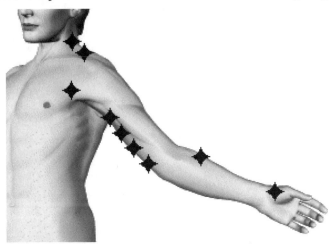

Typical Muscle Spasm Locations, Front

From the front, these are the most common trouble spots where muscles are locked in constant tension to maintain the typing posture and action.

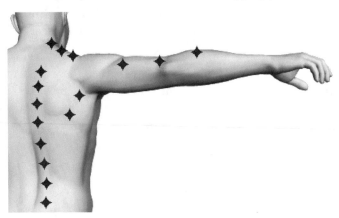

Typical Muscle Spasm Locations, Back

From the back, notice that most of the length of the spine is often in a state of spasm.

Chronic Injury   In the early stages of injury, healing takes place and it is business as usual. But with chronic or cumulative trauma, there isn't enough time for healing to take place completely before another wave of trauma occurs, so the spasm increases. The result is that the accumulated metabolites are not washed away, causing more pain and more spasm, and the cycle continues. Occasionally the spasm compresses a nerve, causing tingling or numbness. Mobility is reduced in the area of the spasm, causing compensation by neighboring body parts that are enlisted for work they are not ideally suited for.

Everyone Has Neck Spasms   Virtually everyone who works at a computer will have muscle spasms in or around the neck. They may be at the shoulder, shoulder blades, or top of the spine. And these spasms are not always problematic; in most computer users, they are a tolerable reaction to the work circumstances, and the total scenario stops short of chronic RSI. For most people, at least in the short term, it just doesn't seem to be a problem, because there are no vulnerable nerves going through those areas.

But for individuals with an unfavorable combination of factors, the spasms are just one link in a larger, damaging chain of events. In our experience, individuals who have muscular trauma paths frequently have specific neck and back spasms. One particular spot is just under the shoulder blade, another runs vertically at the spine. Patients with these spots in an advanced state of spasm are often those who report severe pain elsewhere in the hands and arms. But they aren't always aware of problems in the neck or back.

Test Yourself for Spasms   First try to identify the feel of a healthy, pliable muscle. With your leg relaxed, press on your thigh at the widest spot, about halfway up the leg. Press your thumb into the thick muscle, rolling the muscle as you move the thumb in a circle. Try to find a spot where the thumb easily flattens the muscle and there is no pronounced pain. That's a normal muscle.

Now grasp your forearm at the widest spot (shown below), about two inches from the bend of the elbow. Again, press your thumb into the muscle, rolling the muscle as you move the thumb in a circle. Move around until you find a muscle that "pops" from side to side under your touch as you move your thumb back and forth. That's a spasm. You may have to try this on your upper arm, front and back. Such a muscle is under constant tension, from years of maintaining a static position requiring it to support your hands in front of you. If you've found a spasm, it will be tender and more sensitive to pressure than a normal spot. This is a tender spot.

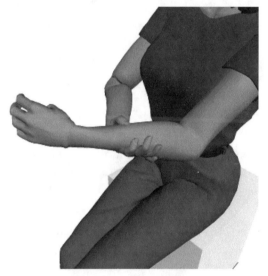

One Spot to Test Yourself for a Muscle Spasm

Press your thumb into the fleshy muscle on the top of your forearm and you might find a muscle that pops from one side to another as you roll your thumb back and forth.

Treatment Strategy for Muscle Spasms

Massage is hands-on therapy for the muscles and fascia, usually administered by a skilled therapist. The goal is to break down muscles that have become locked in a static, unnatural state, encouraging them to rebuild. Massage does this by mobilizing the tissue, increasing blood circulation, and increasing tissue pliability. Massage is more generalized than myofascial release, which also strives to manipulate the ligaments and tendons. Massage is most effective on the arms and legs, whereas myofascial release works best in the neck and back, perhaps because there is less tissue mass.

With the patient lying on his or her back, the therapist should use massage oil or another lubricant to make it easier to roll the fingers vigorously over and into the tissues. The muscles are slowly rolled under the thumb or fingertips, both across the bands of the muscle and then along their length. When going along the length, the therapist usually moves toward the heart, encouraging the waste products of metabolism to flow out of the area. The position of the arm can be changed to expose different aspects to the touch.

When you first start massaging a spasm, the muscle spasms will pop from side to side under your touch. As the spasm is reduced, perhaps after four or five sessions, you will notice a distinct crunching feel, as if several strands of small wire were under your thumb. When the spasm has resolved, you won't be able to distinguish any bumpiness. It will be one flexible mass. For serious spasms, it can take as long as eight weeks to resolve, and more weeks to rebuild healthy tissue.

The process of "spasm breaking" is almost guaranteed to create discomfort initially. This discomfort should start subsiding after three or four treatments. In the meantime, cold packs are a popular choice to reduce the tenderness.

Avoiding Scarring It's important to note that the body heals and rebuilds after massage by creating a certain amount of scar tissue—fibrous, inflexible tissue—and re-molding the prior tissue structures. To minimize the negative impact of scarring, you must perform range-of-motion and stretching exercises throughout your rehabilitation. If you will continue typing after you heal—we presume that's your goal—you will also have to continue stretching exercises after rehab is "completed."

Change Your Habits The causes of the spasms, such as incessant keyboarding, posture, ergonomics, and work-habits, must be addressed so that recurrences can be fewer, milder, and more manageable.

Techniques You Can Use

The following techniques are useful during the early stages of RSI, and also for maintenance, after rehabilitation has been completed. Some relief may be noticed almost immediately, and significant relief often occurs after several sessions. These techniques should be followed by stretches for the sore muscle groups. If the pain increases, the technique is simply not right for you. We must emphasize though, that these techniques, while potentially very effective are not necessarily a replacement for the experienced hands of a good therapist.

As with all exercises and stretches, stop immediately if any of the following techniques cause pain, discomfort, or aggravation of any symptoms.

Neck (Trapezius) Press down on the muscle at the side of your neck, between the neck and the shoulder. This is the upper trapezius, a common tender spot.

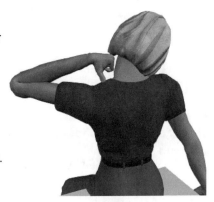

- ❏ Keeping the pressure on the spot, stretch the muscle by tilting your head away from that side.

- ❏ Hold to a count of seven.

- ❏ Do five repetitions three times a day.

Below the Collarbone (Clavicle) Probe for a tender spot below your collar bone. It may be in a depression two-thirds of the way out from the center line to the armpit.

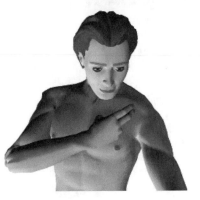

- ❏ Move your arm (on the side you are probing) to various positions to make the spot more accessible… more of a depression.

- ❏ Maintain pressure on the spot while rolling your shoulders front to back through the complete range of motion.

- ❏ Do five repetitions three times a day.

Above the Collarbone Run your
fingers above your collarbone to learn
where its boundaries are. Initially you
will not tend to think of this area as
having any space at all, let alone
freedom of motion. But as you work
your fingertips into the area and move
your arm you will see there is some
space.

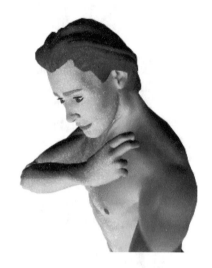

- ❏ With your fingers pressing in,
  move your head and shoulder
  around to see how the space
  opens up in different positions.
  Once you've got some sense of
  the space you can try the
  following mobilization technique.

- ❏ Insert your fingers in the gap above the collarbone toward your shoulder.
  Pull forward gently, very gently… but don't expect any discernable
  movement. Hold to a count of seven.

- ❏ Perform five repetitions three times a day.

Shoulder Blade (Scapula) Around
the border of your shoulder blade (1),
pressure may be applied by another
person or by leaning against a door knob.

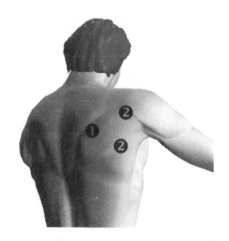

- ❏ After pressure is applied, hold
  your arm out to the side and move
  the arm backwards, keeping your
  elbow straight. This will move the
  shoulder blade back. No hold is
  required for this exercise, but the
  goal is to work through the full
  range of motion.

- ❏ You may also find it helpful to
  massage two spots (2) in the back
  of the shoulder, shown in the
  figure.

- ❏ Perform five repetitions three
  times a day.

Elbow Bend your elbow approximately 90 degrees and point your hand straight out away from you. Probe above your elbow at the back or inside of the arm for a tender spot.

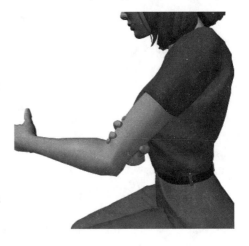

❑ Maintain pressure on it while you flex and extend your elbow.

❑ While maintaining pressure on that spot, turn your forearm from palm up to palm down position.

❑ Perform five repetitions three times a day.

Forearm (Not pictured) With the palm down and the fingers curled, probe for tenderness in the large muscle on the top of the forearm. While maintaining pressure, move the wrist up and down. This technique may be performed with the palm up, with pressure on a tender spot in the upper forearm. Perform five repetitions three times a day.

Wrist (Not pictured) For wrist pain, grasp your wrist with your other hand so the thumb is on the sore spot. Move your wrist up and down while holding firmly on the painful area. Perform five repetitions three times a day.

Thumb (Not pictured) For soreness at the base of the thumb, maintain pressure on the sore spot with your other hand, and flex and extend the thumb ten times. Then move the thumb left to right ten times.

Mid-Back (Not pictured) This combination can help relieve tightness in the mid-back. Lie face down on a bed with your head suspended over the edge, and stretch your neck upward, but not too forcefully. Perform five to ten repetitions. After each set, do a set of five pushups.

Scalp (Not pictured) Scalp massage can be a key to relieving neck and upper back pain. If you probe your scalp carefully, you may find several tender spots. Use deep, circular movements on these tender spots. Repeat as frequently as you feel is helpful.

Resolving Nerve Trigger Points

Where a muscle spasm is in the vicinity of a nerve, especially where the nerve "gives a branch" to a muscle, you may develop a very acute problem spot called a nerve trigger point. They're called trigger points because they elicit symptoms somewhere along the path of a nerve away from their own location. For instance, a trigger point in the upper arm might trigger pain in the hand. A trigger point, when palpated with the thumb will elicit a sharp pain at a very precise spot, somewhat like having a splinter. The pain isn't in any way overwhelming like a sprained ankle, but it can be intense and piercing. *Yet, until you touch a trigger point, you might not even know it's there.*

Note that the terms "tender spot" and "trigger point" are used differently by various sources. We reserve the term *trigger point* for nerve trouble spots, because they trigger pain at other locations. Painful spasms we refer to as tender spots.

Trigger points are, in all probability, areas where fibrous tissue has accumulated on a nerve, tethering it in place. This makes the nerve susceptible to damage from almost any movement because it is constantly being tugged. Instead of slipping and sliding smoothly along its course, it bends, stretches, and rubs. Many therapists have observed occurrences of trigger points on the ulnar nerve in upper arm, and have started to identify consistent locations for them. One particularly common spot is just above the elbow on the inner side of the arm.

Trigger points can be resolved by repeated sessions of deep massage, rolling the thumb or fingers over and into the trigger point, with increasing pressure. With the patient helping to identify areas that are tender, you can zero in on the trigger points rather easily. If you have no access to a good massage therapist, you may be able to administer this technique yourself. Grasp your problem arm between your thumb and fingers, and with your thumb on the trigger point, press in. Roll your thumb in a small circular motion over the trigger point. Flex and extend your problem arm while pressing to create some additional action on the spot.

As with muscles that are in a state of spasm, trigger points will initially pop from side to side under your touch. As they resolve, you'll notice a crackling or crunching texture. When a trigger point is finally resolved, the crunching texture will no longer be noticeable. Go slowly and gently, particularly at first to see what your response is over the course of a few days. Don't assume that pressing harder and eliciting more of a reaction means you are solving your problem faster. There's no way magic rule for how quickly you should expect to resolve your problem spots, but many patients seem to take about two months of massage. Expect to spend weeks, at the minimum. Keep in mind that the trigger point might have formed over years.

When a trigger point breaks through, you may have normal sensation that very instant or starting several days later. We've noticed that it's often not until eight to ten days following the breakthrough that normal sensation occurs. Even if you do get immediate relief, be prepared for other trigger points to come into play after the first is resolved. It's possible that you had two or three trigger points, and relieving the first one frees up your nerve, but only for a short time. Then, like a rubber band that that's being held at several places, the effect of the second trigger point is more noticeable. Although this can be disconcerting, subsequent trigger points can be relieved just like the first. It's also possible that your nerve will simply need a long time to heal at the spot that's been traumatized. We've seen this take as long as four months for chronic sufferers so don't be discouraged if you don't get instant results.

Carpal Tunnel Massage

One form of massage is so unique that it calls for special attention. It involves direct stimulation of the tendons at the carpal tunnel, and its use was reported in an article in the Spring, 1994 Massage Therapy Journal. According to the article, the thickening of the tendons' synovial sheaths, under heavy use, prevents the flexor tendons from moving independently. If you've got this problem, you may be unable to move your pinkie finger independently. You can confirm this by trying to flex your pinkie while holding your other fingers straight. The thickening interferes with blood flow to the nerve, resulting in loss of nutrition to the nerve, and ultimately the formation of fibrous adhesions in the area.

The technique for treating this problem with massage was proven with rowers at the twenty-third Olympiad, as they came back from competition squeezing their wrists in agony. Over the past ten years, one of the Yugoslavia team's trainers had been perfecting the massage technique, called "transverse friction massage" to break up these adhesions, as described in the following excerpt:

"With the athlete's hand relaxed and supported, Petar Ciric would apply deep pressure across the inner and outer aspects of the Olympiad's forearm, just above the wrist. His hope was, by rubbing "across the grain," so to speak, the adhesion points could be broken and the fibrous formations released. This would restore full longitudinal movement to the tendons again, relax the sheaths, and encourage the movement of fresh blood and nutrients to the median nerve, thereby reducing the numbness and restoring grip strength. I had never seen anything like it. It all made sense. The normal therapeutic approach of immobilizing the wrist, applying ice to reduce the swelling, and encouraging rest was exactly what you would do if you wanted to grow adhesive fibrous formations. No wonder these athletes felt worse in the morning when left untreated, or treated with ice therapy."

Rich Phaigh
"Upper Extremity Repetitive Stress Injuries"
Massage Therapy Journal, Spring, 1994

As with all exercises and stretches, stop immediately if the following technique causes pain, discomfort, or aggravation of any symptoms.

To perform this technique, press your thumb into the soft, bottom side of the wrist, one to two inches back from the crease in the wrist. If you relax while you press, you'll notice that your fingers curl toward where you're pressing. Move your thumb around to find the flexor tendons. You have to press fairly hard, but eventually you'll notice your thumb bump over the tendons. Move your thumb back and forth a few times over one tendon at a time, but don't overdo it—this is an intense technique. You can follow the tendons up your arm another inch or two before they become too deep to palpate.

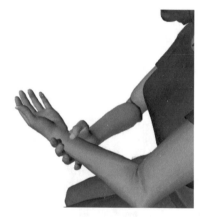

**Directly Massaging the
Carpal Tunnel Tendons**

You can feel and massage the tendons in your wrist by curling your hand to relax it and pressing firmly with your thumb.

You might want to try this technique all by itself, starting off very lightly, *and performing no other massage or other exercises for a few days*. This will help you determine if you react to it positively or not. Remember, it was effective on world-class athletes who had very active, muscular arms and were not in a static posture. Even if it is effective for you, your tolerance for it could be much less.

References

"*Upper Extremity Repetitive Stress Injuries*" by Rich Phaigh
http://hoohana.aloha.net/~billpeay/TECHT08.html
Massage Therapy Journal, Spring, 1994
American Massage Therapy Association

Myofascial Release

Myofascial release is a specific technique of physical therapy that combines aspects of massage, stretching, and joint mobilization to address RSI problems. Its goal is to free up or release tight bundles of muscle ("myo") or connective tissue ("fascia"). The following techniques are used in myofascial release:

- ❑ Gradual sustained pressure on the tight area, combined with breathing exercises.

- ❑ Pressure while stretching along the length of the tissue. This gentle pull is called traction, loosening the length of the tissue, almost like unwinding a knot in a thread.

- ❑ Performing the movement naturally caused by the muscle that needs to be released, while applying pressure to it.

Myofascial release is deeper and more gradual than general massage, and usually targets many of the common tender spots of RSI. The more persistent spots are usually at the base of the skull, between the neck and shoulder, along the inside of the shoulder blade, around your collarbone, behind your elbow, and on top of your forearm. The paths of the nerves in the arm are also targeted because nerve entrapment is often the result of muscle tightness or lack of joint mobility. Most of the massage, stretching, and strengthening techniques that we describe will target the same trouble spots that a myofascial release specialist will emphasize.

Muscle Strength

If you notice difficulty opening jars, carrying grocery bags, opening doors, and so on, RSI has probably affected your muscle strength. In advanced stages of RSI, even coordination problems become apparent. This can include awkwardness fastening buttons, overshooting while shaking hands or picking up objects, and difficulty writing. When muscles become weak they cause joints to become unstable and create imbalances with opposing muscles. This in turn causes other muscle groups to compensate. In extreme cases, muscles gradually forget their function and movements become uncoordinated and inefficient.

Contrast with Endurance Muscle tissue consists of red and white fibers. The red fibers respond slowly to stimulus, but can sustain contraction for a considerable time. The white fibers respond quickly to stimulus, but are unable to sustain the contraction, and fatigue easily. This is the difference between the familiar dark and white meat of poultry. You might not be surprised then, to learn that the two types of fibers have to be trained in different ways. That's why we address strength and endurance separately. In general, strength is easier to achieve than endurance.

How the Muscles are Damaged In an individual with RSI, loss of muscle strength is caused by any of the following:

❏ A progressive reduction of activity, because of the pain cycle, which results in the muscles wasting away (atrophy).

❏ Problems with the nerve that would ordinarily supply the stimulus telling a muscle to contract. This causes reduced stimulation, affecting the muscle's ability to contract.

❏ Formation of fibrous scar tissue which replaces the contractile tissue of muscle. Scar tissue is a particular suspect after surgery.

Early on in the progression of RSI, it can be difficult to decide which one of these factors is causing the decreased strength, so all three are usually considered and treated. Later in the progression of RSI, it is often clear if the nerve itself is the problem.

Strength Is Needed For Static Positions You won't always notice overt signs of weakness. Many RSI sufferers feel just as strong with most mechanical activities, but they have lost a lot of strength in the routine suspension of the arms and upper torso. This makes it hard to work without resting your arms and slouching forward. Muscles perform work even though they're not in motion. This is called a static or "isometric" work, and posture is certainly a prime example. RSI patients often complain of inability to sit for any length of time, and a need to support the head because "the shoulders cannot hold it anymore." So posture presents both strength and endurance problems. Strengthening the musculature is a large part of the solution, but maintenance of a balanced posture also has to be trained.

When to Start Strengthening The goal of therapy in the initial stages is to help the body heal, since the body cannot heal by itself anymore. Usually, when the body has healed to a point where you are mostly pain-free at rest (although the pain may return on activity), you are ready to start strengthening exercises. Increasing your strength should not be done at the cost of increased pain. There's one simple rule: if the strength exercises cause persistent pain, it's still too early. However, note that some soreness is inevitable, just like the soreness that you feel when exercising after a lengthy period of inactivity. By the time strength exercises are initiated as part of your rehabilitation program, you'll probably be capable of distinguishing between the "good" soreness of exercise and the "bad," I-hurt-myself type of pain.

Restore Full Range of Motion While performing a movement, the resistance placed against a muscle, and consequently the strength the muscle must afford, varies based on the angle of movement. Muscles are most efficient and able to exert the most force in the relatively small range of motion used in daily activities. However, to encourage joint mobility and good circulation, it's important to exercise the full range of motion.

Startup Reps As a rule, strength exercises should be increased slowly. *There is no rule that ten repetitions of an exercise have to be performed on the first day.* If you fatigue at fewer repetitions, stop. Do *not* set a goal for yourself and try to complete it regardless of your symptoms. There's no need to hurry since muscles strengthen quickly.

Emphasize the Scapula First Begin with the scapular exercises (described shortly), in which you lie on your back and lift your arms in three positions. Many patients find that the arms feel better rather quickly, whereas the neck and back symptoms linger on, perhaps because they are the first to develop problems. The scapular strength exercises often result in a reduction of symptoms at the neck, provided they are begun at an appropriate time in the therapy. After you've become comfortable with the scapular exercises, you can proceed to the other strengthening exercises.

> "The upper back exercises were key for me. They got my shoulders back in shape so my posture improved."
>
> -- Patient F.

Use of Weights With the arm and scapula exercises, start without any weights. Using weights too early can aggravate your symptoms. After you're comfortable performing about 20 repetitions with each exercise, it's time to include minimal weights such as soup cans. When you can do 20 reps with this weight, you can progress to one-, two-, and three-pound weights. After three pounds, it's up to you. You may want to increase the weight up to five pounds or stay at three.

Exercise Daily Exercises should be performed daily to start off with. Then, as a progression is made to weighted exercises, the frequency may be decreased to perhaps three times per week.

Practice Good Form More important than the weight is to use good form when doing strengthening exercises, so that compensatory movements do not occur. While performing strength exercises without a therapist, watch for "trick" or "substitution" movements where you change the angle of the movement or use a different set of muscles to complete the range of motion for an exercise. Concentrate on the muscles you are supposed to be working. A common example of substitution is when you use the neck muscles to cheat on shoulder movements or other upper arm exercises.

Manual Resisted Exercises (MREs) No exercise can substitute for the value of manually resisted exercises in which a therapist applies resistance to the movement. A highly experienced therapist can work against many of the problems we've described: imbalance in muscle groups, proper range of motion, and coordination. MREs can be the best way to retrain the correct muscle action, while preventing complementary movements. For a patient who has a serious condition and is not perfectly disciplined in conducting his or her own exercise regimen, MREs are the only realistic solution. Only a therapist can modify the resistance based on the strength of the muscle in the different ranges of motion, and adjust the exercises as the patient progresses.

Maintenance As long as the root cause of your problems—repetitive work—cannot be eliminated, your individual battle against RSI will be an ongoing process. Strength exercises should be continued on a regular basis, three to four times per week even after you feel you've recovered.

How Important Is Strength Training?

In our travels across the RSI terrain we learned of a patient who had serious carpal tunnel-like symptoms and made a remarkable recovery under the care of a personal fitness trainer. Anxious to learn his secrets and find out if his techniques were consistent with our ideas, we contacted him and interviewed him at length. The results were quite reassuring. Here's what we found out.

His name is Fred Hahn and he's a Certified Exercise Instructor, running his own company, Serious Strength (www.SeriousStrength.com), in Manhattan. Although not a physical therapist, he's been involved in various aspects of physical therapy for ten years. He worked at New York's Hospital for Joint Diseases and founded and ran a sports medicine practice at Methodist Hospital along with a leading orthopedic surgeon.

The patient in question is a hair stylist, who learned about Fred because she happened to be cutting the hair of one of Fred's employees. She complained of severe aching and burning in her hands and wrists, increasing over the course of a year and a half, until it became incapacitating. If the symptoms were limited to pain alone, she would grudgingly have continued to work through the pain… but when she couldn't hold the scissors in her hand anymore, she was ready to sell her business. She had been cutting hair for 20 years and, being self-employed was an acknowledged workaholic. She described her pain level as "10" on a scale of 1-10. An orthopedic surgeon and a neurologist told her about using ice and other palliative techniques but suggested that ultimately, surgery—carpal tunnel surgery—was her only recourse. Other than the fact that she knew she had had a nerve conduction velocity test, not much diagnostic information was available. (Although this patient is a hair stylist, not a computer worker, what we learn will be just as valuable.)

We asked Fred, "was she physically fit?" thinking of one of the more debatable predisposing factors for RSI—even some very healthy looking people have problems. This is where we dive headlong into Fred's theory and strategy. Irrespective of her overall health, in Fred's view she was not physically fit for the work she was doing, and that's all that matters. All activities are muscle specific, and the muscles that held her arms up and worked the tools of her trade were fatiguing and inflaming. Says Fred: *"Health is substantially a matter of metabolism, and 80% of your working metabolism is from muscle tissue. Disorders that arise from weakness must be countered by strength."* To endure strenuous activity, progressive resistance exercises are critical. Moreover, some of the more popular trends of physical fitness, such as obsessive running, are doing a disservice if they cause you to reduce muscle mass, or even fail to maintain it. Most people really believe that recreational activities keep their muscles strong and healthy. But this is simply not true if muscle mass is slowly decreasing. And the aging process alone will cause you to steadily lose muscle mass, if you don't fight back.

Fred's therapy therefore consists almost entirely of strengthening exercises, and that's how he made her well. Strengthening enhances joint flexibility and vascular efficiency. He strengthened her whole body, her legs, back, and specifically arms. He used a Nautilus biceps curl machine and grip machine, both specially retrofitted for better results. Fred especially emphasizes slow-speed strength training. In this technique, a weight is used that is light enough that the patient can sustain the action for at least 40-60 seconds, but heavy enough to cause momentary muscle fatigue in at most 90 seconds. And note that multiple sets are not performed. Another technique he uses is timed static contraction. With this method the patient holds a weight in a position until complete fatigue occurs. This is what you might know of as "isometric" exercising. Both techniques strive to completely fatigue the muscle in the shortest possible time, with as little articulation of inflamed joints as possible, for the utmost safety.

And how did his client progress? After only three sessions of a half-hour each she started to get significant relief—so much so that she canceled her appointment with her surgeon. She was treated for 17 once-a-week sessions and now has almost no pain. As we've seen with our patients, she had a setback midway through, with an increase in pain believed to be from some strenuous lifting she had done. She's back to working full hours and has given up that wrist brace someone told her to wear. She also has increased the chores she does around the house, which she had greatly curtailed. She continues a regimen of strength training on her own. We said his therapy was *almost* all strength training, so what else does he recommend? He tells his clients to drink one gallon (!) of water a day.

Before evaluating this case history, an important word of caution: this is the story of a therapy for which you will most likely NOT be reimbursed by medical insurance. Fred, like many alternative therapists, is not a physical therapist, let alone a licensed physician. It is not out of the question, however, to have a physician authorize alternative treatment so it can be reimbursed, and insurance situations are changing hourly. The only certainty is probably this: you will only find out what you can get if you fight for it.

So what wisdom can we derive from this therapist's wonderful results? First, we certainly believe it substantiates—and elevates—the value of strength therapy. And, it highlights, from another source, an experience where surgery was one step away, yet apparently inappropriate. The only question is what it implies about other aspects of our therapy, some that you've already read about, and others that you will read about soon: massage, stretching, and ergonomics. In other words, if strengthening alone helped this patient, is that the whole answer?

We believe not. Strength training may have been exactly what this individual needed and was ready for; others are simply not ready. Our experience seems to show that a small number of RSI patients have a seriously diminished capacity for muscle recovery. Some advanced cases don't seem to recover the same strength levels as "normal." They would be traumatized if they start weight training without a chance to reduce their inflammation and aches and pains. Too many patients are put into a "work hardening" program administered by individuals without the expert touch someone experienced in RSI. Fred himself is quick to point out that many practitioners don't have much specific training in how to remodel tissue safely. The other point to remember is that his patient was not a computer pro, but a hair stylist, which almost certainly has more variety of hand motions and postures.

Differences aside, we feel Fred's success speaks volumes. Here's how we put it in perspective: in contrast to massage and stretching which will help *heal* damage that has already been done, strengthening (and ergonomic changes) will help *maintain* your health—keeping you less susceptible to damaging yourself again.

References

Fred Hahn, Serious Strength
www.SeriousStrength.com
169 West 78th Street, New York, New York 10024
(212) 579 9320

Muscle Endurance

The capacity of a muscle to sustain prolonged activity is called its endurance. RSI sufferers will usually have both weakness and fatigue symptoms, so it's important for a therapist to explain the difference between the two to the patient, since endurance is slow to increase. It's not unusual for the process of improving endurance to continue for six to twelve months or more after the patient has been discharged from rehabilitation. This slow return to your prior level of endurance is one of many frustrating aspects in the RSI healing process.

Another consideration is that endurance is very activity specific. Many of us know this phenomenon from skiing or other sports that we only occasionally partake in—we're extremely sore after just a few hours of skiing for the first time each year. This means that just because you might be able to vacuum two rooms without any increase in symptoms, it does not mean that you can necessarily wash a car. Each new activity has to be trained, and as you recover from RSI, you are essentially rebuilding your muscle mass. What were once very familiar activities are once again new to your body. As you exercise to restore your endurance, you must be aware of what your body is telling you and avoid overdoing it. This is an aspect of RSI recovery that therapists particularly need to instill in every patient.

Repetitions Versus Weight Muscle strength and endurance go together, but strength is quicker to progress. Only increase weight resistance after establishing some progress with endurance at each level. A good guideline is that once you can do three sets of ten repetitions for a given exercise, the weight may be increased. Each time a progression in weight has been made, drop the repetitions down to what you can accomplish, and gradually work up to three sets of ten again. For example, work with a one-pound weight until you can do three sets of ten. When this is comfortable, increase the weight to two pounds, but drop back the repetitions to one set of ten. In time, work the repetitions back to three sets, and increase the weights again.

Some exercises are more difficult than others—don't force yourself to advance just as rapidly with every exercise.

> "I had good success doing the "lat raise" exercise. It's a weight machine in which you lift weights with your elbows. It really improves the shoulder muscles. I could only do about 30 pounds when I started, but was surprised how rapidly I got up to 70… a likely indication that I had lost a lot of capacity over the years. I worked up to this by doing three sets of ten. When I could do three sets of 13, I moved up ten pounds and dropped back to 10 reps."
>
> -- Patient E.

Record Your Initial Capacity Make a serious effort to get baseline information when you start exercising. Especially with exercises for the hands and arms, where you can compare one hand to the other, you can get very revealing diagnostic information. When you first try the various exercises, do them once or twice until exhaustion, and write down your results. Remember, you only have one chance to get baseline information… once you start exercising, your circumstances change.

> "I started doing wrist curls with a 3-pound weight and could do about 60 before my left hand was completely exhausted. Then I tried my right and was surprised to find after 200 I could keep going, almost as if I had no limit. No wonder my left hand has nerve problems."
>
> -- Patient E.

Time Your Working Fatigue Cycle When you are typing and using the mouse, time how long it takes you to fatigue or have pain. Then, the next time you're typing, try to take a break before you reach that limit. Over a period of time, you can try to gradually increase that time slowly, a few minutes at a time. Your tendency will be to forget about your limits and increase the continuous keyboarding time until the discomfort returns. The key is not to flirt with disaster, but rather, to be very in tune with your body's changing capacity and stay within your limits. The idea is to stop *before* fatigue happens.

Aerobic Exercise Aerobic exercises, also called conditioning exercises are fast, high-intensity activities that get your heart pumping and your lungs working. They're extremely important because they increase blood supply to inflamed body parts, which is vital in the healing process. Another healing benefit of aerobic exercise is that it reconditions your overall sense of vitality and endurance. Because of your RSI, you've probably become somewhat de-conditioned, and not just in the parts where you feel symptoms. The body as a whole needs to regain strength and endurance. Aerobic exercises should be started early in the rehabilitation program. It can consist of a variety of activities including a stationary bicycle, walking on a treadmill, jogging, or "aerobics" programs. And you should definitely continue some aerobic exercise as part of your routine after your rehabilitation has been completed. But don't get so obsessed with aerobics that you end up decreasing your muscle mass. As we learned earlier, you need that muscle mass to provide strength and boost your metabolism.

Returning to Work and Play   If you've persevered through an arduous rehabilitation or post-surgical period, you'll probably have to relearn many skills and build up your endurance again. Some people may also be returning to a workstation that has had ergonomic improvements while they were away from work, recovering. So it will be normal to experience fatigue and discomfort. Listen to your body… when you're tired and achy, rest and stretch. Gradually things will get better.

If you have stopped activities such as gardening, handiwork, or hobbies because of your symptoms, when you are ready and you restart, your symptoms may recur. Don't get discouraged. Stop when your symptoms occur, but gradually, over days, weeks or months, increase your activity in small increments.

If you've been out of work, your rehabilitation may include what is referred to as "work simulation" before you return to work. Here you actually simulate your work conditions and practice your work activities. Be warned, however, that the first time you sit at a computer workstation after a period of time, it is going to be rough. You may not be able to make it through the first five minutes, but as days go by, you will see improvement. Just make certain that you work only at a workstation that is completely adjusted to your individual specification.

Strength and Endurance Exercises

You might not feel that you are lacking in the strength department, but it's very likely that your muscles have lost a lot of vitality and some are in a state of spasm. Strengthening exercises have three objectives:

To improve the "carriage" of your head and shoulders, to get them back over your spine so your chest is not pulled taut by your neck. As you work on this, you don't want to end up in a state where you are constantly tensing your shoulders to pull them up. Instead, you want to get to a point where your shoulders are habitually back, but relaxed, falling comfortably at your side.

To increase the stamina of your arm muscles, particularly the small muscles involved in constant typing.

To change your muscles from their fibrous, ligament-like quality, back to the resilient quality of active muscles.

As with all exercises and stretches, stop immediately if any of the following techniques cause pain, discomfort, or aggravation of any symptoms.

Lying Down Arm Lifts (Scapular Exercises)

This set of exercises will encourage your shoulders to move back, by increasing muscle tone at the back of the shoulder blades.

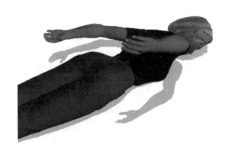

❑ Lie down on your stomach, on the floor or in bed, with your arms down at your side.

❑ Lift your hands up off the surface. The most they might rise is about a foot. Hold 3 seconds, and lower.

❑ Repeat 10 times, and 3 sets.

❑ My initial count _____.

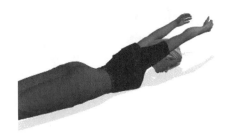

❑ Now move your arms up over your head, straight in line with your body. Point your thumbs up. Again lift your hands up off the surface. Hold 3 seconds, and lower.

❑ Repeat 10 times, and 3 sets.

❑ My initial count _____.

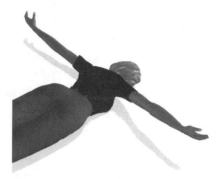

- ❏ Next, hold your arms at a 90-degree angle to your torso, like a big cross, again with your thumbs up.

- ❏ Again lift your hands up off the surface. Hold 3 seconds, and lower.

- ❏ Repeat 10 times and 3 sets.

- ❏ My initial count _____.

- ❏ As you improve your strength, try each position with small weights then gradually increase the weights. Holding even soup cans in your hands can make a big difference.

"Lat" Raise

If you have access to a gym, one of the most effective shoulder exercises is the 'lat raise." This is a strong section of the body, even if you don't consider yourself a powerhouse. If your shoulders have been drooping, you will probably feel a difference in your posture after as few as four sessions.

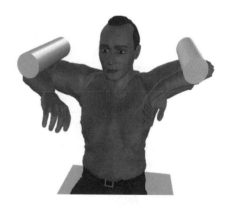

- ❏ In the lat raise machine, you sit down and place your arms out at your side, under padded bars, with your hands in toward the center.

- ❏ You then "flap your wings" upward, like a chicken, lifting weights.

- ❏ Try 3 sets of 10 with a very easy weight setting. You should be able to increase your weight fairly easily after just a few sessions.

- ❏ My initial weight: _____ and repetition _____.

Seated Lifts

This exercise is important because it counterbalances the force on your shoulders, keeping the shoulder joint in better alignment. Over the course of time, the muscles *below* the shoulder become very weak, adding to the imbalance that moves the shoulder forward.

- ❏ While seated on a stable, firm surface, lift yourself by pressing down with your hands. You may have to place small pillows under your hands to lift more comfortably. If your hands hurt, curl the fingers and use your knuckles. Alternatively, push up on your elbows, using several pillows.

- ❏ Hold for a ten count if you can.

- ❏ Repeat 3 times. Gradually increase the duration over time.

- ❏ My initial count: _____.

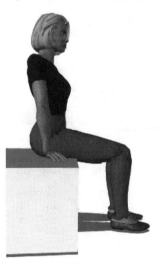 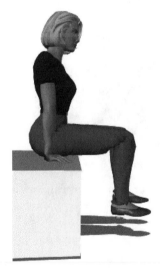

Wrist Curls

This set of exercises improves your stamina for holding your hands over the keyboard.

- ❏ Hold a small weight in your hand and, if necessary, rest your forearm on a horizontal surface, such as the large arm of a comfortable chair or your lap. Your palm should face the centerline of your body.

- ❏ Lift the weight by bending only your wrist, not by raising your arm.

- ❏ Do 3 sets of 10.

- ❏ My initial count _____.

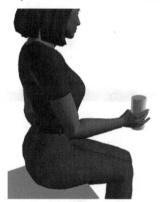 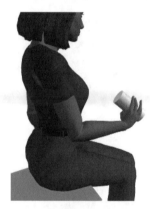

- ❏ Now turn your palm **down** and repeat 10 times, again lifting upward.

- ❏ This time turn your palm **up** and repeat 10 times, again lifting upward.

- ❏ With your palm still facing up, move the weight **left-to-right**, from the wrist.

- ❏ Do 3 sets of 10 for each position.

- ❏ My initial count _____ / _____ / _____ / _____ .

Rubber Band Around All Fingers

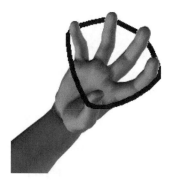

- ❏ Get a rubber band that forms a circle of about 4 inches, and is approximately 3/8" wide. (Good ones are often available on fresh produce such as broccoli or asparagus.)

- ❏ Put it around the tips of all of your fingers and the thumb of one hand.

- ❏ Widen your fingers to stretch the rubber band outward. If it's too hard to do, or the rubber band is just too large, find one that is better or put a binder clamp on it to make it smaller.

- ❏ Repeat opening and closing until you reach your limit, such as the first signs of fatigue, pain, or the inability to perform slow, controlled movements.

- ❏ My initial count _____.

Rubber Band from Thumb to Finger

With the same rubber band, wrap it around your thumb and just one finger. You might need to wrap it an extra time around the thumb to take up the slack.

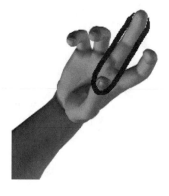

- ❏ Extend the finger, stretching the rubber band.

- ❏ Repeat opening and closing until you reach your limit.

- ❏ Repeat for all four fingers.

- ❏ My initial count _____.

Flexibility and Stretching

Flexible muscles are like rubber bands, in that they stretch to allow the range of motion required for various activities. Muscles that have diminished flexibility due to lack of movement, lack of exercise, or scarring, are vulnerable to even more damage. Inflexibility has numerous repercussions:

It prevents joints from working through the complete range of motion, and can create a "catching" sensation during certain movements, such as reaching out for something.

Inflexibility can contribute to "pulled" muscles, which subsequently cause mis-aligned joints.

Inflexibility encourages compensating use of other muscles, possibly causing your symptoms to spread.

Inflexibility can cause micro tears in muscle fibers when you move, resulting in scarring, inflammation, and a further decrease in flexibility. In other words, once you get your muscle accustomed to being in a static position, it is a snowballing phenomenon.

A normal part of the aging process reduces the moisture content of your tendons, ligaments, and connective tissue, and as these fibers become less flexible, they shorten, binding everything together more tightly. Remember that, unlike most of the body's other cells, your connective tissue does not replenish itself by constantly dividing into new cells… what you have is what you've got! If you insist on performing repetitive motion tasks all day into your fifties, these tissues are going to need all the encouragement you can give them.

The primary weapon in the battle against inflexibility is stretching, one of the most important first steps of RSI treatment. Stretches gradually lengthen tight muscles and nerve. (Connective tissue, on the other hand, is not believed to stretch.) This increases your range of motion and flexibility so that these tissues are in a relaxed, unconstrained state when you work. Initially, stretching a muscle that has been relatively static will cause generalized discomfort. This is because of a marked increase in fluid and cells sent to the area as part of the healing mechanism. This discomfort subsides in a week or so, if the stretches are performed consistently.

Resistance, Not Pain   It is important that you stretch to the point of resistance, not pain. If you feel pain when you're stretching, then you're stretching too much, so ease up a little bit. Be gentle during stretches; tissue elongates with frequent gentle stretching. Gradually, you will notice an increased range of motion and increased ease of stretching.

Keep in mind that you may have this RSI condition in the first place because you are susceptible to overdoing things... don't apply the same obsessive, all-or-nothing mentality to stretching!

Duration Each stretch should be held for approximately seven seconds to start off. Then, as symptoms subside, increase the hold to about 12 seconds. Concentrate on deep breathing and relaxation during the stretch.

Frequency Stretches should be performed frequently throughout the workday. We recommend two or three exercises (different ones matched to your symptoms) every half hour, initially. After you start to feel some increase in flexibility, you can increase the interval between stretching to 45 minutes or an hour.

Favorite Stretches You will develop favorite stretches and will find yourself doing them more often. That's fine since the final stage of your management of RSI is for you to recognize your symptoms and be able to control them. So, if a particular stretch feels right, and you want to do it more often, go ahead. Just don't ignore the other body parts for days at a time.

> "The neck stretches really help me. When my symptoms flare up I tilt my head to the side, then roll it forward and backward. I'll even pull gently to the side with my hand. I get immediate relief from this."
>
> -- Patient F.

Maintenance Just as with strengthening and endurance exercises, you might guess by now our final recommendation: stretches are a way of life... you must continue doing stretches as long as you continue to work at your computer. Even at home, whether painting, gardening, or doing other physical work, performing stretches will make the activity more comfortable and improve your tolerance for computer work.

*As with all exercises and stretches, stop immediately if
any of the following techniques cause pain, discomfort,
or aggravation of any symptoms.*

Arms Behind Back

This stretch will help increase the space
for the nerves across your chest area at the
thoracic outlet and brachial plexus.

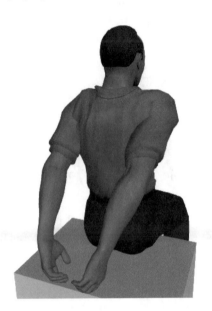

- ❏ Sitting on a bed or other surface
  without a back, hold your arms
  behind you and try to touch your
  hands together. Keep your elbows
  straight.

- ❏ Now try to lift your arms upward.
  Your progress can be measured by
  how high your arms can extend
  while touching your hands together.

- ❏ Hold for 7 seconds.

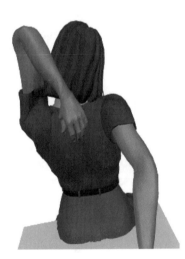

Elbow Up In The Air

This stretch increases the range of motion of
your elbow, upper arm, and shoulder.

- ❏ While standing up or sitting, extend
  your arm straight up into the air. Then
  with your hand, reach down behind
  your back to the center of the shoulder
  blades. Try to push your elbow back
  while keeping it high in the air. You
  can even pull your elbow toward the
  head with your other hand.

- ❏ Then try to reach farther down your
  back.

- ❏ Hold for 7 seconds.

- ❏ Repeat with the other arm.

Arm Across Chest

This is another stretch for your upper arm and shoulder.

❏ Extend your arm in front of you, parallel to the ground, and bring it across your chest, pulling on the elbow with your other hand.

❏ Hold for 7 seconds.

❏ Repeat with the other arm.

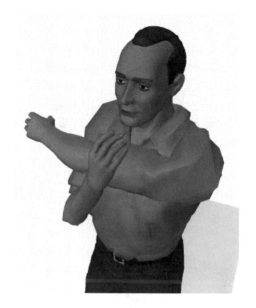

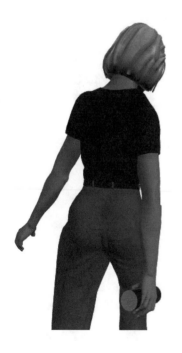

Arm Pulled Down by Weight

This stretch will help create some mobility around the shoulder. You can do this one standing up or sitting down.

❏ Hold an 8-10 pound weight in your hand, and simply let the weight hang at your side.

❏ Hold the weight for about 10 seconds and then put it down.

❏ Repeat 3 times.

Pronator Stretch

This stretch loosens the pronator muscle, the one at the inside of your forearm that can pinch nerves between the elbow and wrist.

❑ While sitting or standing, rest your arms down by your side, then raise your forearms in front of you parallel to the ground. The palms should be down, just as if you're about to use the keyboard.

❑ Then rotate your thumbs, counterclockwise for the left hand, clockwise for the right hand. Rotate them until you feel a comfortable stretch.

❑ Hold for 7 seconds. Repeat with the other arm.

❑ Make a mental note of how far you can rotate your forearm. Observe whether you can increase this range of motion over the course of several weeks.

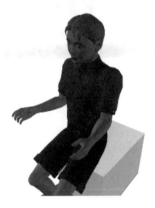 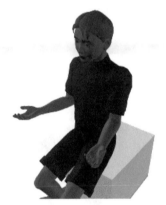

Scalene Stretch

This exercise stretches the two vertical muscles at the front of the neck, that go roughly from the collarbone area to deep under the chin.

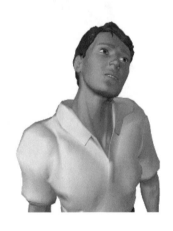

❑ Tilt your head to the side, and then, while tilted to the side, tilt it back.

❑ Adjust the position until you feel resistance from the muscles in the neck.

❑ Hold for 7 seconds.

❑ Repeat, tilting to the other side.

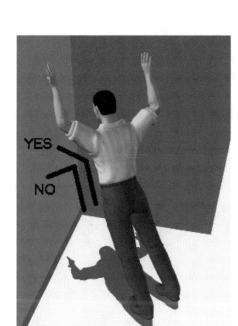

Chest Stretch

This one stretches the pectoralis muscles, which can press on the nerves as they pass through your armpit.

❏ Hold your arms up at both sides and, bending at your elbows, rest your forearms against two walls forming a corner.

❏ Now let your chest and torso fall forward, but make sure your neck is relaxed. Adjust the stretch by moving your upper arms at a 45-degree angle. At the proper angle you'll feel a strong stretch across the chest.

❏ Hold for 7 seconds.

Neck Stretch

This stretch can relieve the tension that accumulates around the neck.

❏ While seated or standing, pull your head straight back without tilting it.

❏ Hold for 7 seconds.

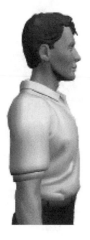

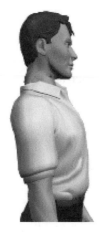

Wrist Stretch

This stretch helps improve your range of motion at the wrist.

- ❏ With your left hand straight out in front of you at arm's length and your elbow straight, bend your hand up so that your palm is facing away from you.

- ❏ Then pull your palm back with your right hand.

- ❏ Hold for 7 seconds.

- ❏ Repeat with the other hand.

- ❏ Repeat with the hand bent down, palm still facing away from you, pulling your palm toward you.

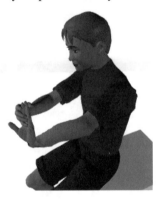 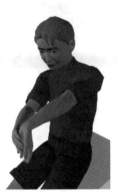

Lower Back Stretch

This stretch works the piriformis muscle deep in the pelvis area, an area that is especially tight from sitting all day long.

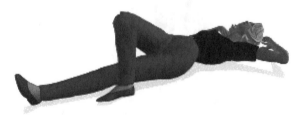

- ❏ Lying down, fully extend one leg.

- ❏ Cross the other leg over and place the ankle against the outside of the extended leg's thigh. For some added stretch you can pull the knee across your body a little more by pulling with the opposite hand.

- ❏ Hold for 30 seconds.

- ❏ Repeat with the other leg.

Back Stretch

This stretch helps improve the flexibility of your back.

- ❏ Lie with your back flat against the floor.

- ❏ Bring your knees to your chest and hold with your hands.

- ❏ Hold for 30 seconds.

- ❏ Slowly release, returning your feet flat on the floor in front of you with your knees bent.

- ❏ Repeat 3 times.

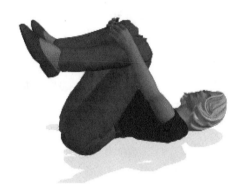

Back Stretch- "Camel and Cat"

This is another stretch to improve the flexibility of your back.

- ❏ On your hands and knees, collapse your back and raise your head up high.

- ❏ Hold for 7 seconds.

- ❏ Now arch your back like a cat and drop your head.

- ❏ Again, hold for 7 seconds.

- ❏ Repeat 3 times.

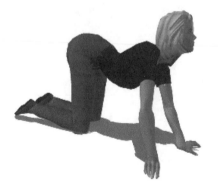
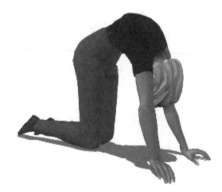

Finger Stretch

Technically, this is called the "interossei" stretch, meaning between the bones of the hand.

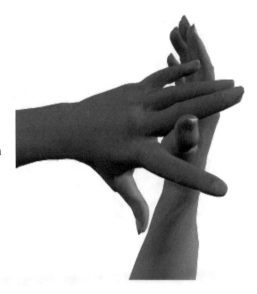

- ❏ Hook your left thumb against an immovable object like a table or doorknob. Gently pull each finger away from the thumb. Make sure you hold the whole finger and not just the tip while stretching.

- ❏ Hold for 7 seconds.

- ❏ Repeat for each finger.

- ❏ Repeat with the other hand.

"I think I've identified one particularly tight spot... muscle tightness across my chest. I've been doing the stretch where I stand in a corner with my arms up and lean into the corner until I feel the stretch across my chest. Originally when I tried this I didn't notice anything... no stretch, just resistance. Then after a few weeks, I tried again and was more patient, and there it was, a very pronounced stretch, achy but a good feeling. In retrospect, I probably couldn't achieve the stretch in prior attempts because I was so tight across the chest."

-- Patient E.

Nerve and Tendon Glides

Glides are movement exercises, without any resistance or exertion, in which you move your arm or hand from one position in which a nerve or tendon is on its shortest path to another position where it is on its longest path. Ideally, in the case of a nerve glide, the nerve starts out slack and ends up somewhat taut, thus providing a gentle, back-and-forth tug that helps free it from points where it is trapped or impinged. Glides also try to lengthen a nerve that has shortened or lost its elasticity from lack of movement.

Nerve Glides These are exercises specifically for the nerves, so their greatest value might be for patients with nerve trauma. However, they also work well in situations where muscle tightness causes nerve compression, as is the case with thoracic outlet syndrome. Nerve glides probably work best if you have a moderate, not severe, state of trauma. In other words, if you have strong sensations of numbness and indications of very sore trigger points that have not been substantially softened or "resolved", the nerve might not be free enough to glide. In such a case, trying a glide may simply provide more tension at the trigger point. On the other hand, if the nerve is only moderately pinched—perhaps you feel pins-and-needles—or it is under pressure from an inflamed muscle, the nerve may glide and these exercises can help. You simply have to try them to find out.

Nerve glides are intended to be used whenever you are working, at the instant you start to experience nerve symptoms such as pinching, pins-and-needles, or numbness. In addition to the stretching action, they provide a respite from your continuous, static work position if you use them routinely. Although glides are an on-the-spot technique, they're more than just a palliative so you should also use them as routine preventive exercises.

Try seven repetitions of each glide whenever you start to feel sensation problems. Stop your work to do them. If the glide is effective, many patients will feel an improvement in sensation at that very instant. If so, we're not suggesting that you've "cured" yourself but you have identified the nerve in question and shown that your situation is controllable to some extent.

Use the following diagram to help you decide which nerve glide might be most likely to help, based on which fingers have symptoms. If fingers controlled by both nerves are affected, emphasize the brachial plexus glide since both nerves go through that area.

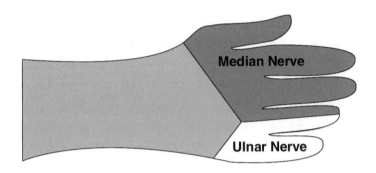

Distribution of the Nerves among the Fingers

This figure shows that the median nerve innervates the three big fingers and half of the ring finger; the ulnar nerve innervates the other half of the ring finger and the pinkie.

As with all exercises and stretches, stop immediately if any of the following techniques cause pain, discomfort, or aggravation of any symptoms.

Median Nerve Glide

The median nerve goes to the index and middle fingers, half of the ring finger, and the entire thumb, but there are some variances among individuals. Try this exercise if you experience nerve symptoms in these areas.

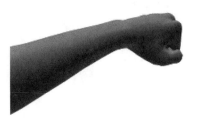

Position 1

1. With your left hand in front of you, palm down, start with a gentle fist, wrist bent down.

2. Open and splay your fingers. Extend your wrist.

3. Simultaneously turn your palm upward. Try to turn your wrist as far counterclockwise as you can.

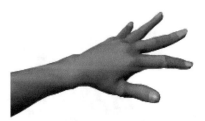

Position 2

4. With your other hand, reach under your hand and grab the base of your thumb. Gently pull downward, trying to extend the rotation a little. Make sure to pull from the base of the thumb, not the joints.

5. Repeat 7 times.

6. Repeat with the other hand.

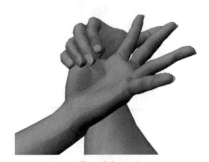

Position 3

This glide resembles the motion a magician makes showing you there's nothing in his hand.

Ulnar Nerve Glide

Your ulnar nerve operates your pinkie finger and the half of the ring finger that is near the pinkie. Try this exercise if you experience nerve symptoms in these areas.

1. With your arm level to the ground, put your right arm straight out to the right. Your palm should face the ceiling. Tilt your head away, to the left.

2. With your head still bent, twist your forearm (from palm up to palm down) through its full range of motion.

3. Repeat 7 times.

4. Repeat with the other arm.

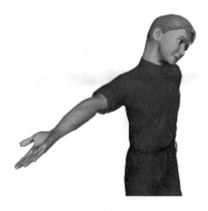
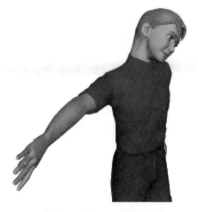

**Ulnar Nerve Glide,
Beginning Position**

**Ulnar Nerve Glide,
Ending Position**

*You'll really feel the action of this glide exercise in your forearm.
If it's too intense, raise your arm up at an angle.*

Radial Nerve Glide

Your radial nerve controls muscles in the upper arm and forearm, and is responsible for the sensation of the top of the forearm and part of the top of the hand. Try this exercise if you experience nerve symptoms in these areas.

1. Let your right arm hang down by your side. Twist your wrist counter-clockwise so your palm faces backward. Bending only your wrist, lift your hand to the rear.

2. Lower your right shoulder down toward the ground and tilt your head away, toward the left.

3. Return to the neutral position, with your arm hanging loosely by your side and your shoulder and neck relaxed.

4. Repeat 5 times.

5. Repeat with the other arm.

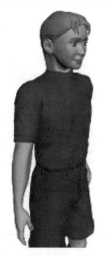

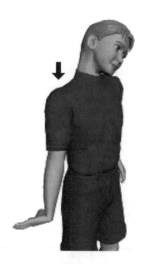

**Radial Nerve Glide,
Beginning Position**

**Radial Nerve Glide,
Ending Position**

Make sure to get your shoulder and neck into this motion.

Brachial Plexus Glide

This exercise enhances the mobility of the nerves at the neck, chest, and armpit areas.

1. Start with your right hand rolled to a gentle fist, tucked under your chin. Your arm should be by your side with your elbow bent as much as possible. Tilt your head toward the right.

2. Then un-bend your elbow and fingers and simultaneously stretch your arm all the way out to the right. As you do so, bend your wrist the opposite direction of the previous position and splay the fingers. Reach back behind your body as well as you can.

3. Simultaneously tilt your head the opposite direction.

4. Repeat 7 times.

5. Repeat with the other arm.

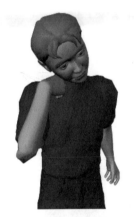

Brachial Plexus Glide, Beginning Position

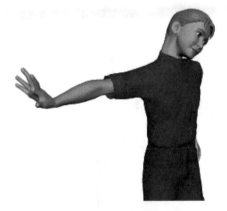

Brachial Plexus Glide, Ending Position

Think of the whole motion resembling an overly theatrical goodbye wave.

After a little practice you should be able to make a nice flowing, ballet-like movement out of it, getting your neck nicely involved. If you notice crackling in your neck, ease up… don't swing your neck as vigorously or as far.

Tendon Glide

This exercise employs the same gliding stretch technique, but this time it's for the many small tendons and muscles that control the fingers.

1. Hold your hand in front of you, palm facing toward you. Bend all of your fingers simultaneously, but just at the two joints farthest from the palm. They should form fishhooks, but not curl into a fist. Try to emphasize your form in this beginning position, keeping your first knuckles very straight and bending both joints as close to 90 degrees as possible.

2. Hold for five seconds.

3. Then move your fingertips down to the middle of the palm. Hold for two seconds.

4. Finally, move the fingertips down to the pad of the palm, press against the pad and hold for two seconds.

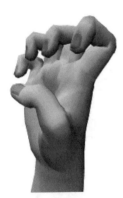

**Tendon Glide,
Position 1**

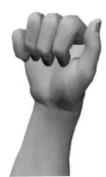

**Tendon Glide,
Position 2**

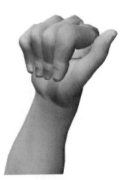

**Tendon Glide,
Position 3**

This glide can loosen up your fingers and relieve the tension on the tendons that flex them.

Improving Joint Mobility

Movement that occurs at the joints is constrained by muscles, connective tissue, and the anatomical configuration of the joint itself. Computer-related RSI often reduces joint mobility due to any of three contributing factors: scar tissue, tightness of fascia or muscles, and fibrous tissue buildup called adhesions.

❑ Scar tissue is usually a result of surgery at the specific spot of an operation, so it's a relatively straightforward suspect after surgery.

❑ A therapist can recognize tightness simply by the feel of the muscles. Muscle or fascia tightness is caused by unequal application of the muscles during computer use and from the compensation pattern as the disorder progresses. You won't directly feel the imbalance that occurs from years of holding your arms in one position… you'll only feel the damage that it eventually causes.

❑ Adhesions, and to some extent scar tissue, can both result from inflammation and what would otherwise be a healthy repair process.

Whatever the source, the net result is a joint that feels stiff and cannot achieve its full range of motion. As with so many of the RSI factors, stiff joints start out being purely a result, but become a contributing factor that causes other problems, such as compression of nerves and blood vessels. Some joint mobilization techniques can be performed on oneself, but this is an area where the most effective treatment is by a therapist. Since joint movement is controlled by muscles, the primary therapeutic techniques are the muscle stretching and strength exercises that we've already covered, along with the following additional measures.

Heat, Massage, and Stretching   Muscle and fascia tightness can be reduced with heat, massage, myofascial release, and stretches. Scar tissue and adhesions should be loosened with massage and myofascial release. For inflammation, physical therapy modalities such as ultrasound and iontopheresis may be considered if the inflammation is not too chronic.

Cold Packs   If inflammation is present, the exudate, which is a product of the inflammatory process, can be reduced with cold packs.

Joint Mobilization Exercises   Joint mobilization consists of moving a single joint back and forth, all the way through its range of motion. It may be performed by a therapist with or without active participation from the patient. Both options can be effective, although in more advanced cases, active participation from the patient is preferred. The following joints typically need mobilization:

- ❑ **Shoulder** Overuse of the muscles on top of the shoulder causes the muscles underneath the shoulder to become weak. This can cause "clicking" or "catching" of the shoulder when you move. Shoulder mobilization is done by a therapist with repeated circular and back-and-forth movements of the whole arm, usually with the patient lying on his or her back.

- ❑ **Collar Bone** The nerves emerging from the neck and going to the arm are often trapped in the neck's scalene muscles and underneath the collar bone. Although the collarbone does not move much, even under good conditions, it can be given a little room by pulling gently behind it and using pressure below it.

- ❑ **Upper Arm** Most of the muscles that move the wrist originate from the elbow area and tightness of these muscles may cause poor joint mobility at the elbow. The tight areas are often resolved with the myofascial release technique of traction and simultaneous pressure, but the elbow often needs joint mobilization to restore its full range of motion.

- ❑ **Wrist** Wrist mobilizations are extremely helpful in achieving relief of symptoms. Similar results are obtained with mobilization to the joints of the hand. With the amount these areas are used during computer work, imbalances are often very pronounced, with the wrist sometimes permanently contorted. Because the bones and muscles in these regions are so small, any tightness, combined with the incessant forces of typing can cause instability. This is manifested as "cracking," pain, or tenderness. Joint mobilizations, followed by stretching and strengthening exercises help reinforce correct position and movement patterns.

> "Suparna was able to restore the freedom of motion to my shoulder blades by doing lots of mobilization of the arms. Then she strengthened my arms and shoulders by placing resistance against my arm while I lifted in various directions."
>
> -- Patient F.

Managing Pain

Not all RSI patients experience pain—some patients instead have varying forms of numbness or incapacity—but when pain is present, the nature of it varies widely. The pain could be achy or sharp, localized or generalized, constant or intermittent, burning or throbbing. For some, pain occurs only during specific activities... for others it is so unrelenting that it governs their lives. When present, pain usually becomes the primary focus of treatment.

Be Prepared for Ups-and-Downs Having chronic pain sends your body into physiological cycles that make it difficult to heal without careful management. The goal of treatment is to break these cycles and allow the body to start healing. Typically, when RSI pain returns after some initial success in reducing it, it is with the same intensity as before. This can be frustrating since you would expect the pain to decrease in intensity. However, in our experience, it is usually the *frequency* of discomfort that diminishes first. So you will notice that there are times in the day that the pain is tolerable or unnoticed, but then it peaks again. Being prepared for this can reduce the frustration. Gradually, the peaks are not as high and you will have gentler ups and downs. Toward the end of your treatment, you'll experience fewer ups and downs. By this time, you'll have become more aware of what your body is trying to tell you, and you'll be better able to manage the symptoms.

Relapse Before Therapy Ends Many RSI patients who are treated by a therapist notice an increase in symptoms just before being discharged from rehabilitation. This is difficult to explain but could be attributed to fear of being on one's own, and the resultant increase in tension. It's a good idea for therapists to warn patients well in advance about this phenomenon. If the exacerbation occurs without warning, patients can suffer from feelings of loss of control and unpredictability, which increases the anxiety and results in a worsening of the physical symptoms. Again, knowing what to expect can be a key to coping. Understanding the basics of RSI is vital to managing it, more so than with many other injuries.

Treat All Pain Seriously Although pain is subjective in that its effect on individuals varies, it is no less serious than other symptoms. If pain is present, it must be taken seriously because it is often a signal of potentially serious deterioration later on. Pain will trigger other reactions in the body, causing cycles of avoidance and compensation that make your RSI factors snowball. Therefore, if pain is not managed early, it becomes increasingly difficult to resolve.

Don't Treat Pain "In a Vacuum" Personality and psychological factors play an important role in the manifestation of pain, so behavior modification becomes as important as the anatomical and ergonomic aspects of RSI treatment. Consider whether your overall stress level, satisfaction with your work, and energy level (or lack thereof) are contributing to tension that aggravates your symptoms or makes you less tolerant of pain. If so, address those factors as genuine root causes of your RSI.

Medications Are Temporary Various pain medications can be effective, but you must recognize that they serve only to treat the symptoms, not the causes of your problems. The effect of medication is only temporary if no treatment to the root cause is provided. We believe that anti-inflammatory medicines are helpful in the initial stages of RSI, perhaps the first few months, but are ineffective in more advanced stages.

Pain Modalities Several "pain modalities," meaning technological devices such as electrical nerve stimulators, can be used by therapists to control your pain. As with medicine, pain modalities are temporary but may help you get through particularly uncomfortable times. As importantly, they can give you a chance to establish better habits without as much avoidance of painful areas and the resultant compensation. In moderate to severe cases, pain modalities do not provide any long-term relief, but they can help with residual symptoms. Our experience indicates that TENS units (described shortly) often have good results for muscular trauma paths.

Ice and Heat Ice is used successfully by many RSI patients and to some extent may be effective for its numbing effect. It is generally useful for reducing inflammation, and will be effective against pain that is caused by muscle inflammation. Heat can be useful for throbbing, achy pain. Experiment to find out which is best for you. Some find that alternating between hot and cold is helpful. Although wrist rests are not a mainstay of our overall theory, there is one model, Case-Logic's Gel-eez®, that is gel-filled and can be frozen or warmed. Some patients get good results from TENS units along with ice or heat when pain flares up.

TENS Units

Transcutaneous electrical nerve stimulators (TENS units) are battery-operated devices the size of a pack of cigarettes, that you attach with wires to your skin in the vicinity of an area of pain. They cost about $100 and are available through physical therapists and doctors. This is a palliative of sorts, since it doesn't address the root cause of the problem causing the pain, but it can be an effective part of therapy for individuals in considerable pain.

The basic principle is that a TENS unit sends a pulse of electricity at regular intervals, which activates your nerve to a slight extent. This releases endorphins, the body's normal response to pain, and causes a counteractive influence that subdues your sensitivity. In other words your nerve gets a little overloaded and you don't notice the pain.

Usually, TENS units are helpful for patients who have muscle inflammation and not so helpful for those with nerve problems. This is because inflammation causes genuine pain which is sensed by a properly functioning nerve. Nerve problems, on the other hand, are due to trauma of some sort that makes the nerve's performance erratic, but not necessarily inflicting constant pain. Nerve problems are also more likely to fade away when not typing so there is less need for a palliative. For such patients, the pulsing of the TENS unit might simply be another nuisance sensation.

References

Gel-eez® Wrist Rests
Case Logic Ergo Products
http://www.caselogic.com/computer/ergo/index.html

Posture

Collapsed posture is one of the main factors of the RSI syndrome. Computer users often have rounded shoulders and their head pushed forward. There are many causes for poor posture, including anatomy and personality factors, but the major culprits with RSI are fatigue and poor workstation configuration. Sitting for hours on end at a computer, holding your head up and your arms suspended out over the keyboard inevitably causes fatigue of the neck and mid-back muscles. Consequently, the shoulders roll toward the chest and the head moves forward. This causes the front neck muscles to tighten, including the scalene muscles, which can pinch the nerves and blood vessels to the arm.

Sitting for any length of time with little movement puts tremendous stress on the low back. Remember, as we explained earlier, that a change in one part of the curved shape results in dangerous compensation in the others.

Try this little experiment: While sitting in a chair, deliberately round your low back, pushing it backwards. Watch how your head moves forward and your shoulders get rounded. Now sit up, erect at the low-back. Notice that your head retracts. The significance of this is that you must treat the entire spine as one big system.

Balance Is the Key What is "good" posture? The human body has a natural alignment, where the body is under the least stress, and the musculature is not excessively tensed. The key to this low-tension position is balance: your upper torso and head are balanced over the mid-torso and lower back so they rest on top of one another and don't require muscle tension to hold things in place. Correcting your posture will have to be done slowly and with determination. Be gentle while correcting your posture. Don't try to pull your shoulders as far back as possible... the goal is balance, and minimum tension. In the correct position, your spine has the natural curvature, your chest is "open," meaning that the shoulders are back a little, so they are centered on the plane of the torso. Even when standing, pay attention to the poor habit of standing with your abdomen protruding... concentrate on pulling your stomach back a little.

Associate Posture with an Activity Don't try to think about your posture constantly throughout the day. Instead, select an activity that you do frequently and periodically, and check on your posture at this time. For example, every time you answer the phone, notice your posture. Then forget about it until the next time you answer the phone. Gradually, the constant reminder will help you maintain the preferred posture.

Get Moving One key to good posture is to maintain the proper alignment during movement. Good posture does not mean holding a single position for a prolonged period of time. The human body needs movement. Only in movement do the muscles contract and the joints move, facilitating blood flow and the subsequent nourishment to your body parts. Movement becomes essential to maintaining balanced posture, because if there is no movement, the muscles fatigue easily.

Use a Good Chair Make sure your chair provides good support and encourages the proper curvature of the spine. Because of poorly sized chairs, many women are forced to sit too far forward. Even sitting properly puts a lot of stress on the spine, and sitting without support is worse. Make sure the seat pan is not so long that sitting all the way back is uncomfortable. Conversely, taller individuals need chairs with a longer seat pan and higher back. It's very common to need more lower back (lumbar) support than most chairs offer. Try putting a rolled up towel in the back of your chair to see if you are more comfortable. If it seems to help, specially designed lumbar supports, such as the inflatable one from Medic-Air (see References at the end of this section), are available that attach to your chair.

Avoid Armrests   We recommend resting your hands in your lap when you're not typing. If you must rest your arms on the chair armrests, make sure they're low enough that they don't cause a shrugging action at your shoulders. Use of armrests is not recommended while you are typing.

Posture Education: The Alexander Technique   If you feel that poor posture is a serious problem for you, there are a number of specialized disciplines devoted solely to generalized awareness of body form. The Alexander technique is just one example. F.M. Alexander was a Shakespearean performer who was plagued by voice loss. To solve his problem, he set up mirrors to observe himself as he recited, and discovered that as he recited he contorted his body quite dramatically, and generally became very tense. These observations led him to discover a connection between underlying patterns of tension and how this affects our activities. He went on to develop the Alexander Technique, a unique system for self-management of bodily stress. You can investigate the Alexander technique and others on the web or in the Alternative Medicine Yellow Pages.

Check Your Eyesight   If you haven't had your eyesight checked within a year, do it now. All the best ergonomic measures won't be effective if you invariably lean toward the monitor to compensate for incorrect vision.

References

The Alternative Medicine Yellow Pages
http://www.amazon.com or your local library
Future Medicine Publishing Company
98 Main Street, Suite 209 Tiburon, CA 94920

Jenny Adler's Web Page on the Alexander Tecnique
http://www.ozemail.com.au/~herbandjenny/index.html.

Medic-Air Back Pillow and Lumbar Roll
http://www.novicom.com/ptp_medicair.htm

Vision

As we touched on in the previous section, if you strain to see the monitor, you'll probably contort your posture either forward or backward. If your vision might be a problem, we could take the expedient route and recommend glasses or contact lenses. Instead, we strongly suggest that you investigate the topic of eye exercises.

In the course of writing this book, we investigated the topic and were somewhat startled by what we read. In a book written by four M.D.s in the vision field, we read a continuous theme that echoed almost exactly the message that we've formulated on behalf of your arms. The book is *Improve Your Vision Without Glasses or Contact Lenses* by Steven M. Beresford, et al. In it we learned that the traditional medical community fixates on mechanical solutions and crutches, instead of delving deeper for root causes and addressing them. The following poignant analogy is drawn between glasses and other injuries: if a doctor, after putting your broken bone into a cast, told you that you'd have to wear the cast for the rest of your life, you'd limp out of the office yelling and screaming. Yet that is exactly the prescription we casually accept when we visit the optometrist. Why?

By traditional thinking, poor eyesight is caused by genetically inheriting poorly shaped eyes that eventually don't work so well. But doctors have known conclusively since at least 1968 that we develop poor eyesight because of an emphasis on close work. This has long been the case because we do so much reading, and as you may imagine, has increased with our increased computerization. If you're interested, the conclusive information is from studies on communities of Eskimos that have a long track record of excellent vision. Yet when their children attended our schools for the first time, their vision suffered exactly in proportion to industrialized children.

You may be so accustomed to your glasses or contact lenses that you would understandably dismiss this theory as questionable, maybe even "crackpot." But if we also told you that, according to this theory, your reliance on corrective lenses predisposes you to eye disease such as glaucoma and cataracts later in life would you be more motivated to act? If their theory is right, even the newest laser surgery techniques, which apparently are having wonderful results, are not the healthiest of options. That's because they allow you to persevere without restoring the vitality of your eyes' musculature and blood flow.

Briefly, their theory is that your focusing capabilities are controlled by muscles, not the flexing of the lens or the immutable size of the eyeball itself, and these muscles must be deliberately worked. Note that they are not by any means alone in this theory—their work appears to be based on extensive pioneering by William H. Bates, M.D., as long ago as 1940. The gist of the therapy consists of six focusing exercises. Your results certainly will depend on how bad your eyesight is, but some people experience results in as little as a month.

References

Improve Your Vision Without Glasses or Contact Lenses:
A New Program of Therapeutic Eye Exercises
by Steven M. Beresford, 1996

Reducing Habitual Muscle Tension

Is tension a cause or an effect? We use the term tension in the mechanical sense, referring to the pull on muscles from both ends, rather than the more figurative sense of life's stressful demands on you. For that, we reserve the word *stress*. Constant or excessive muscle tension is the enemy. It could certainly be exacerbated by external stresses, but in our experience, the most important stress on most computer pros who get RSI is from within, an irrepressible passion for their work. Perhaps the source is an intense concentration level called for by the problem-solving nature of computer work... or perhaps it's the long, uninterrupted sessions of work. We just don't know for sure.

Whatever the direct or indirect sources of your problems may be, it's the intolerable degree or frequency of muscle tension that delivers the damage to your system. Ultimately all of the therapies and techniques that we recommend strive to get you to work without your muscles in a state of constant, damaging exertion. Some techniques aim to achieve less tense positions; others will attempt to rework your body to loosen tight areas. One way or another you must reduce the cumulative level of muscle tension.

Breaks

Taking breaks from your work might be the most significant and most challenging change to make in your work habits. And, despite its low-tech nature, it is the most universally agreed upon recommendation from all authorities on RSI. Advice varies greatly on the right amount of break time and frequency, and there is no right answer, considering that there is no substantiation behind the advice. There is only good sense combined with experienced judgment. Here's ours:

How Long Should Breaks Be?

Our quick guideline on breaks: Take a 2-5 minute break every 15-30 minutes of work.

Take mini-breaks every 3-5 minutes, where your hands leave the keyboard and touch something else that causes you to move your entire arms.

If you type whole paragraphs or successive lines in continuous sessions where your hands are at the keyboard without your arms changing position, you need breaks. Your arms must entirely change their alignment so the intertwined braid of muscle, nerve, and bone unlocks itself and breathes. Your muscles must un-tense, so they don't fatigue and inflame. The precise, correct timing is unknown. The more frequently you rest, the better. If you can stop every ten minutes for a one-minute break, where you genuinely reset your tension level, that may work for you. Others suggest five-minute breaks every 20, 30, or 60 minutes, but we think 60 is too long. Only you can judge for yourself. Here are some additional ideas:

- ❑ Taking breaks does not have to mean stopping work. Instead of emailing someone, walk to their desk.

- ❑ If you're simply gathering your thoughts, don't hold your hands poised at the keyboard. Instead, stand up, stretch, walk around, get a drink of water.

- ❑ Place a reminder program on your computer, that comes to the foreground automatically every so often, reminding you to take a break. It will take some discipline to pay attention to the reminder and stick to the schedule. If you find you are ignoring it, increase the interval and decrease the duration to a combination that you can start to honor. Then try to gradually shorten the interval.

- ❑ As a classic type-A personality, you would probably do well to find ways to use breaks as a productive technique, since you might be physically incapable of actually taking a break. Print out articles from the Internet and go off for a walk to read them. Our favorite site for this is Macmillan Publishers, mcp.com. They have full versions of many current computer books, and you can download any five at a time in your "personal bookshelf." Or visit and learn about your co-workers and their accomplishments.

References

The Reminder, by Steve Kellock, text only
http://www.silversoft.com/reminder/

Stress Away Break Reminder, with graphics
http://www.stressaway.com/

Vergo Personal Break Reminder, animated
http://www.vergo.com/

Macmillan Publishers
Downloadable books to read during breaks
http://www.mcp.com

Exercise While Sitting in Your Chair

Many simple exercises can be performed while sitting in your chair to break the tension that results from being locked in one position. Here are a few techniques you can use.

- ❑ Do pelvic tilts, rolling your pelvic area backward as if flattening your lower back against your chair, then back to the neutral position. This can alleviate low back stiffness.

- ❑ Stretch your neck, head, and upper back. Slowly roll your head in circles.

- ❑ Shrug your shoulders up and down and then roll them in circles.

- ❑ Hold your hands behind the back of your chair and stretch your chest muscles.

- ❑ Get your feet moving with simple leg exercises like marching, kicking, and ankle pumps (raising and lowering your heels).

- ❑ Stretch your fingers frequently.

- ❑ And don't forget our glide exercises.

Seated doesn't have to mean sedentary!

Breathing

Computer users often develop a subtle, but distinct habit of breathing very shallowly and using only the uppermost part of the chest to breathe. This cheats the body of oxygen and contributes to the overall phenomenon of tightness in the chest area, because the upper chest muscles become strong and tight. Breathing is an unconscious or "involuntary" function but you can improve your breathing habits when seated at the computer, with a conscious effort. Improvement starts with an understanding of the three types of breathing, which are distinguished by the muscle groups that contribute to the effort:

❏ Apical, which takes place at the apex of the lung (top portion of the chest). Your chest and shoulders rise and fall when you are doing apical breathing.

❏ Intercostal, which takes place from the rib cage. Your chest expands like a balloon when you breathe intercostally.

❏ Diaphragmatic, or abdominal breathing, which takes place below the rib cage. In this type, your belly moves in and out as you breathe.

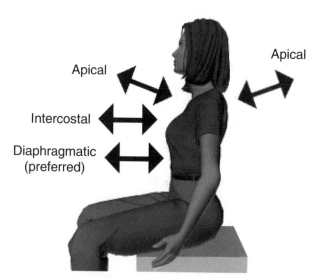

The Three Types of Breathing

The figure shows the three areas that can dominate your breathing. Apical breathing, with short breaths, is common when seated for long periods.

Practice exaggerating each type to feel the difference. Ideally, all three breathing patterns should contribute to each breath. When you're at rest, your breathing should be mainly intercostal and diaphragmatic. RSI sufferers emphasize apical breathing because the sedentary, monotonous, seated posture encourages it.

There is another whole theory on RSI that attributes the entire problem, in a way, to breathing, or rather the lack of it. In his book, *The Mind Body Prescription: Healing the Body, Healing the Pain*, Dr. John Sarno describes what he calls "tension myositis." By this theory RSI and many other chronic pain syndromes such as back pain are directly caused by low oxygen flow to the muscles and other tissues. And what causes the low oxygen flow, you may ask? According to Dr. Sarno, it is from various psychological factors including but not limited to suppressed anger (he uses the term *rage*), anxiety, low self-esteem and so on. Depending on how you interpret it, the tension myositis theory borders on the "it's-all-in-your-head" theme so offensive to most RSI sufferers. But we think the broader message *does* fit in with our explanation of RSI, even if your only psychological problem is a compulsive concentration on your work. To that extent, you must free up your mind, relax your chest, exhale deeply, and get moving so your blood gets flowing. Don't just sit there locked in one position, with an increasingly focused attention to the keyboard… so much so that your muscles themselves don't breath.

In our section describing our case study patients, we described one patient, Chris, who obtained only partial success with our regimen. Now that we've introduced the *Mind Body Prescription*, here's the rest of Chris's story:

> "The stretching, massage, and improved ergonomics didn't solve my problems. There was more to it than that. I was treated by Dr. Sarno, who diagnosed me with tension myositis syndrome, his name for the complex of pain that is ultimately caused by unresolved emotional conflicts. After attending his seminar and getting considerable help from a psychotherapist referred by Dr. Sarno, I've made more progress. We determined that my problems were caused by traumatic issues related to family life and my career. I'm back to typing almost as much as before… I still have some symptoms but I'm in control. And my workstation is much different than in the past… everything is adjustable and set at the right position… and I use voice recognition software."
>
> -- Patient C.

Dr. Sarno's theory is that many deep-seated, unresolved conflicts of modern life are inevitable and now epidemic. The brain manipulatively brings these traumas to the surface by manifesting them as physical pain... as an outlet or shunt against the alternative of dealing with them emotionally. But enough of the psychology—what does this mean to RSI sufferers? This patient's experience lends credence to the notion that psychology can be at the root of RSI problems, but the relationship is still difficult to clearly map out. If emotional trauma is the whole answer, then Chris could go back to typing full-time, ignore positioning and breaks, and not be at risk. Unfortunately, we're not optimistic that that is the case. We suggest that emotional problems are simply one additional fuel on the RSI fire, not tremendously different from oppressive work schedules, sleep deprivation, aging, or a poorly configured workstation.

Use the following strategies to improve your breathing habits.

Abdominal Breathing It's important to consciously emphasize abdominal breathing to relieve tension from the chest muscles. To practice abdominal breathing, take a deep breath through your nose while inflating your abdomen. Actually push your belly out to get in the habit. Exhale through pursed lips. This simply creates a habit which emphasizes fully exhaling. Consciously relax your upper chest and front neck area. This emphasis on abdominal breathing is also important when you are doing strengthening exercises.

Breaks One of the most difficult aspects of maintaining your recovery will be the challenge of filling your break times with activities other than typing. One convenient solution is to use breathing exercises to add some variety. Every once in a while, use your break to count ten or twelve abdominal breaths. You'll see it's also a relaxation technique.

References

The Mind Body Prescription:Healing the Body, Healing the Pain
Dr. John E. Sarno Warner Books 1998

Keyboarding Techniques

If you work at the keyboard all day, you may need to make quite a number of changes to your habits. These may initially frustrate you, but like everything else, your body will gradually learn these new techniques and they'll start to get easier. The following techniques are some of the most important elements of our therapeutic strategy. Don't discount—or worse, dismiss—them because they aren't flashy, or don't involve cutting flesh, or a quick fix. Remember, it took you years of working in an habitual, detrimental fashion to completely overwhelm your body's substantial capacity for self-rejuvenation. Try to accept the logic of recommendations that point to equally cumulative changes in the way you work.

Use Large Muscle Actions The most important change you must make involves the way you move your hands from one key to another. Instead of keeping your lower arms stationary, moving and stretching only your fingers to reach the keys, get your whole arm moving. Move your shoulder and upper arm a little bit to contribute to the motion. This will result in much less bending at the wrist. And it will use the muscles of your upper arms and shoulders, rather than the smallest muscles, the ones in your lower arm that power the fingers. If you've shown signs of a predominantly muscular trauma path, this emphasis on large muscle movements is vital because the large muscles of the arm and shoulder are less prone to fatigue.

Don't Reach Out Sit with your elbows close by your side, not out far in front of you. The idea is to avoid having to hold up the weight of your arm any more than necessary. If your arms are in close, with your elbows near your body, the upper arms hang down without any force required to keep them suspended. The difference is shown in the following figure.

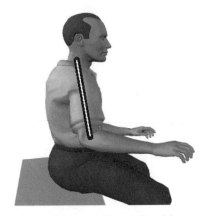 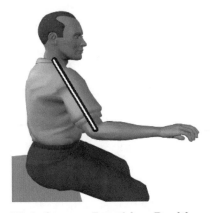

Low Stress, Close Position	**High Stress, Reaching Position**
With your arms in close, less weight is suspended.	*Reaching out like this requires your shoulders to work all day long.*

The more you reach out in front of you, the more lifting force it takes to hold your arms up... and the more tension is produced. One issue that this borders on is the question of what angle to keep your elbows at. Many sources suggest that your elbows must be at a 90-degree angle, but we don't think it's as simple as that. There is probably no perfect angle… ideally you should stay in motion. Nevertheless, we do prefer a somewhat "open" angle, meaning greater than 90 degrees. The important thing is to find a comfortable position that minimizes muscular exertion.

Avoid Single-Handed Combination Keys One way to avoid small muscle actions is to change the way you do combination keystrokes such as Control-S or the infamous Control-ALT-Delete. (Will we someday start our cars by pressing Control-ALT-Delete?—Let us pray not.) If you are very strongly conditioned to use certain combination keystrokes, consider removing the Control or Alt key that you use the most. On most keyboards, the keys easily pop off with a screwdriver. We've found that the left side Control key is one of the most frequently used combination keys, so you might consider removing it first. This will force you to use two hands to do those combinations. If you haven't had problems related to use of the mouse, you can certainly consider substituting mouse techniques for combination keys. However, if your situation has many indicators of a generally reduced level of tolerance for repetitive work, beware of shifting an unbearable workload from one trouble spot to what will simply become a new one.

Two-Finger Typing If you have severe muscular symptoms and you're a fairly fast (translation: "*compulsive*") touch typist, you should consider—at least initially—typing with just your index fingers. This is understandably a very difficult transition for any typist. If you can't justify such an extreme step, at least train yourself to move your arms more when you reach to the numbers on the top row of the keyboard. Then try to do the same for the keys that require the most stretching of the pinky fingers. If two finger typing clearly helps you, you may decide to try transitioning to the next technique, six-finger typing, after you prove that you can control your symptoms for a significant period of time.

Six-Finger Typing A less restrictive option is to type with only three fingers on each hand. For an experienced touch typist this will initially be just as inefficient as hunt-and-peck is for new typists, but over the long haul, not as much of a compromise as two-finger typing. The value is that it eliminates the pinky fingers. This is important because the pinky fingers use the smallest of the small muscle bands, and they are involved in motions that are the most contorted. Make sure if you use this technique that you move your hands and arms… don't just twist your wrist to compensate.

Keep Your Wrists Comfortably Straight The motion that you make with your palms facing down, when you slide your left hand toward the left or right hand toward the right (shown in the following figure), is called ulnar deviation. It's called ulnar deviation because the motion is toward the ulna, the smaller of the two forearm bones. When you type, avoid bending your wrists, side-to-side, to reach the keys. Instead move your forearms a little.

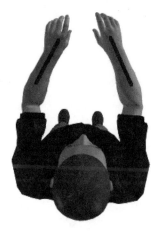 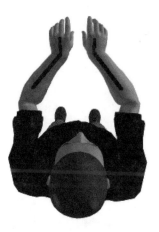

Normal

This position causes less irritation in the wrist.

Ulnar Deviation

With your wrists bent, every keystroke can rub the tendons in your wrist together.

Ulnar deviation is widely implicated by many RSI theorists, as a cause of tissue irritation, and it only makes sense. The nerves, tendons, and blood vessels that course through the small carpal tunnel surely must be more constricted or abraded when you bend the wrist outward. This is substantiated not so much by formal studies linking cause and effect, but from the personal experiences of RSI sufferers. Some longtime RSI sufferers have symptoms that are so pronounced that they can turn them on and off by certain actions such as ulnar deviation, as if throwing a light switch. Try your own test… hold your hands at their most ulnar-deviated position and do some make-pretend typing with all ten fingers. You may find that you can't go a full minute before the outside of your forearms start to burn.

Use a Gentle Touch Use a light touch to strike the keys. If you've ever noticed that you can hear some vigorous typists from quite a distance, you can understand the excessive force they're exposing themselves to. Are you the same??? Keyboards are available that reduce the force needed to strike the keys. Get one on a trial basis. And keep your fingernails short—long fingernails make typing more strenuous by making the action more deliberate and causing an odd angle at the last finger joint.

Use Fingers, Not Thumb on the Spacebar   Avoid hitting the spacebar with your thumb. Instead, try to move your entire arm back and hit the spacebar with your fingers. A surprising number of RSI patients report aggravation of the thumb, and the way they hit the spacebar is a likely cause.

Change Slowly   Do not try to make these changes all at once. The mere act of changing, even to the most favorable configuration imaginable, is stressful because you must concentrate on the new habit. With the stress comes tension. To start with, change just one or two things at a time, or try them for five minutes out of every hour. As it becomes easier, increase to ten minutes, and so on.

Persevere   If you do get frustrated with these new techniques, don't give up too quickly. Yes, it will be hard to know how long to persevere... because results will not be so quick that you can easily correlate success to specific techniques. If a technique seems to make sense to you give it at least a few weeks.

Voice Recognition Software

One of the most effective ways to reduce muscular tension in your arms is not to use them. And only very recently, voice recognition software has improved to the point where it is a realistic alternative to typing. In fact, substantial portions of this book were "typed" with voice recognition. Although it's not perfect, we believe this technology has certainly passed the point of what's called a breakeven. In other words, it saves enough time to justify the nuisance of learning it. Voice recognition software now allows you to talk at a normal speed and use everyday language to tell your word processor what to do.

We originally tried one of the lesser-known names in voice recognition software with unsatisfactory results. It would constantly pick up background noise no matter how it was adjusted. And it didn't seem to be accurate enough, missing too many words. IBM's ViaVoice, for $40, produced much better results. The background noise situation was controllable and the accuracy was unquestionably better. But make no mistake about it, this is not an instant solution. Even ViaVoice still picks up some unintended noises. The phrase "Then we bought IBM's..." was originally transcribed by ViaVoice as "Womb that what IBM's tumor." Be prepared to invest at least a few weeks training the software about your voice and acquiring enough proficiency to reach your own personal breakeven. *Learning all of the techniques is the key!* You may find it unsuitable to use in a cubicle, but some of our case study patients have not found this to be a problem, since you can speak very softly to dictate.

The other top voice recognition program is Dragon Dictate's Naturally Speaking. The leading programs all seem to routinely "leapfrog" one another for the lead in the technology, and are alternately chosen by different reviewers as the favorite. Check the latest reviews to find out which one is currently leading the pack.

References

"Computing Out Loud," Voice Dictation Web Page
http://www.out-loud.com/

Toxins and Diet

Coffee, alcohol, cigarettes, sugar, pollution, you name it. Our bodies are essentially one big filter that copes with all the things we ingest out of habit or force. Exactly how this impacts the RSI patient is the subject of much discussion but little concrete information. By the account of Dr. Ray Wunderlich, RSI is substantially the result of technology and Twinkies (his thesis, our words). He postulates that poor diet, characterized by highly processed food, is substantially responsible for RSI problems.

While we don't agree with the Twinkie theory, we do accept the simple logic that toxins reduce your tolerance for repetitive work because they devitalize your health. They sap your body's innate healing powers by using up water to filter the toxins out... water that would otherwise be used to moisturize, lubricate, and wash metabolic waste products away from aggravated tissues. You must decide how heavily you think this plays into your RSI strategy. Some suggest that megadoses of various vitamin and mineral products are helpful, but we're doubtful. Others say that sugar products bind glucose to your connective tissue and gum up the works... we'll wait for better information. Many people are convinced that increasing their water intake is helpful. Among the many possibilities, this is one that is hard to argue with. You can't go wrong by increasing your water intake substantially.

> "I've made a habit of drinking a glass of water first, every time I get coffee, and I only get a half-cup of coffee. It's been an easy compromise and cuts back on the coffee because I'm not as thirsty."
>
> -- Patient D.

References

The Natural Treatment of Carpal Tunnel Syndrome:
How to Treat 'Computer Wrist' Without Surgery
Ray C. Wunderlich., Jr., M.D. 1993, Keats Publishing.

Rest

The worse your problem, the more important sleep might be. During sleep your batteries are recharged and your body's natural healing powers get their chance to do their thing. The more time you give it, the more chance it will have to fulfill its mission. When you're not well rested, the tendency to fatigue is increased. Your shoulders fall forward more quickly, starting the litany of complications. And the small muscles in your arms fatigue more quickly from the constant, repetitive tension, causing the inflammation that eventually leads to the dangerous pain cycle.

There's no magic to judging your own sleep needs... listen to your body. Force yourself to get enough rest. For instance, don't stay up at night writing books about your problems (!). If you are challenged by family responsibilities, compensate by resting whenever you can, even if it's not at night.

Melatonin You may want to check with your doctor and try melatonin pills to improve your sleep. Although recent studies contest its efficacy, the theory is that it replaces a chemical that you produce less of as you age, one which regulates sleep at night. Fibromyalgia, that cousin of RSI, is strongly associated with a reduction of the deepest periods of sleep. Whether it is a cause or effect of fibromyalgia is unclear, but there is reason to suspect that the most valuable recuperative effects of sleep only occur during the deepest phase of sleep. Generic melatonin, available from any pharmacy, may help you get that deep sleep you need.

Mattress Pad   If you repeatedly experience numbness in your hands at night, your problem might be that your nerves are being pinched against your mattress, under the weight of either your arms or torso. One potential solution is a one-inch-thick foam mattress pad that contours more closely to your arm, and therefore reduces the pressure at any point of contact. Such pads are now available that are made from a material called visco-elastic foam, which has a very adaptive consistency, so it molds to your shape.

Yoga

Yoga is starting to get increased recognition for its ability to combat RSI. If you believe that an overall tension level has set the stage for your particular situation, it makes sense that yoga can help. In fact, one of our patients decided to pursue yoga more seriously, and has found it to be so rewarding that she's since left the computer world to be a yoga instructor. More on her experience after we explain yoga in our own words.

For our purposes, yoga is almost synonymous with *concentrated relaxation.* We'll explain some basics if you want to get an idea what it's all about and experiment with it a little. In full regalia, yoga can be a lifestyle. But we feel that you can invest in yoga to any extent. If you find the mere idea of ritualized relaxation somewhat rubbing against your grain, then— ironically—it's probably just the medicine for you. In other words, your lack of capacity for relaxation is specifically the problem. You are relaxation-challenged.

Try this simple exercise. Lie down on your back on a comfortable floor. Listen to your breathing. Starting with your fingers, make a conscious effort to relax them—*tell each finger to relax,* one at a time. Then tell your hand to relax.... then your lower arm... and so on up your arm. Next, repeat for the other arm, legs, and parts of the torso. You may become aware that some parts were tense when you didn't even realize it. The point is to consciously develop an awareness of what relaxation means to each part of your body.

Another technique, involving breathing, is explained in the book *Recovery Yoga,* by Sam Dworkis. The simplest exercise is just to concentrate on your breathing. Lie down and try to count your inhales and exhales for three straight minutes. You don't necessarily have to count them, you can simply listen to and feel each breath, but counting is the easiest way to convey what you're trying to do. You'll almost certainly find your mind start to wander well short of your goal. In fact, you may find this to be an excellent technique to fall asleep; that's not a failure… simply a sign that you're able to deliberately control your ability to relax.

If you suspect that general tension, and perhaps poor oxygen flow to your muscles is a likely description of your scenario, you would do well to investigate yoga. This is exactly what one of our patients did:

How One Patient Battled RSI with Yoga

Alice had been typing for over ten years when she developed chronic RSI symptoms, primarily what we've called a muscular trauma path. She had reached the point where pain in her hand, arm, and neck was so debilitating it forced her away from her job, managing software developers. After four doctors and two therapists failed to help her, she was diagnosed by Dr. Pascarelli and treated by Suparna. To make a long story short, she got significant relief from the therapy we've spelled out—she estimates 85 percent—but in the course of the journey decided that the underlying work/life style was less than it should be. Here is her message about RSI and yoga:

"Yoga literally means 'union' of the mind, body, and spirit. According to the Sivananda philosophy of yoga, to unite the three, one must engage in the necessary practices of: exercise, breathing, relaxation, diet, positive thinking, and meditation. The combination of these items, *when done properly,* has a profound effect on the mind, body, and spirit. In the West, the mind, body, and spirit are treated as separate entities that are not connected. For example, we go to a doctor to mend our bodies, a house of worship to attend to our spirits, and a psychiatrist to heal our minds. In the East, the mind, body, and spirit are not only interrelated, but inseparable; disease is considered a signal of blocked energy resulting in a physical manifestation. In the East, it is impossible to talk about disease without considering the state of the mind and spirit.

"Yoga can benefit RSI sufferers in many ways. Most have been sitting in front of a computer for years. Their bodies have become tight and stiff, stress has battered the areas where computer use is concentrated, breathing has become shallow and irregular, and muscles and tendons have worked so hard to keep the body in this position that they have actually shortened. Hatha yoga concentrates on stretching and strengthening the entire body, teaching correct breathing (full diaphragmatic, intercostal, and apical breathing), learning deep relaxation, and quieting and calming the mind. By practicing yoga over time, the body becomes more supple and capable of relaxing.

"On a physiological level, the yoga practitioner consciously and unconsciously learns how to decrease the stress in the mind and body and increase the ability to relax during daily life. In doing so, he or she learns to inhibit the "fight or flight" response—the sympathetic nervous system—which to this point has been over-activated, and activate the "rest and repair" response, or the parasympathetic nervous system, which has been underutilized by the body. The response of the nervous system directly affects proper breathing, daily exercise, calming the mind, and genuine relaxation.

"It takes a long time to repair injuries incurred over a long period. When RSI patients begin to pursue yoga, they may find themselves in relapse and reinjury because yoga requires using all parts of the body including the main RSI trouble spots. The first time I did yoga after having numerous RSI symptoms for two years, my hands and arms were so out of shape because of injury that I could not do major portions of the class. I could not use my hands to support my body; I used my forearms and elbows instead. In addition, it changed me mentally—I wanted to do the postures. When I pushed myself, I found myself in pain that often took considerable time to heal. Over and over again, I learned patience. It took a long time but eventually, I could do a whole class using my hands. When I was strong enough to complete a class, I learned through pain that I still had little endurance. Some of the yoga postures are very repetitive and I am still prone to injury resulting from repetitive motion. I suspect that many RSI patients will experience the same.

> "Attending yoga classes also taught me that my mind ran uncontrollably, and that I was unable to relax. There is a time to rest between postures and at the end of the class. Over time, I learned what relaxation really means. It took me a long time to understand that I was not relaxing and that my mind was not calm. Meditation was also a key for calming my mind and enabling me to relax.
>
> "For RSI patients, the process of rehabilitation brings body awareness, emotional awareness, and soul searching about the presence of the injury. By relaxing the body and calming the mind with yoga and meditation, the RSI patient soon experiences the body becoming more supple, and comes to a more peaceful understanding of their injury. As in any activity, RSI patients must be careful in their practice of yoga, learning their body's limitations, and accepting them. With time and dedication to yoga, you can heal your repetitive strain problem."
>
> -- Alice Bell

This former patient is now teaching yoga, and we encourage you to contact her to help with your situation, whether RSI-related or not.

References

Alice Bell, Yoga Instructor
(212) 929-4798
bellap83@hotmail.com

Recovery Yoga; A Practical Guide for Chronically Ill, Injured, and Postoperative People
Sam Dworkis, 1997 Three Rivers Press
www.randomhouse.com

Biofeedback

Biofeedback is the technophile's alternative to yoga. It is the electro-mechanical way of training your body to understand and attain a relaxed state. Biofeedback is a technique where your brainwaves are detected and displayed (or indicated by sounds) so you can recognize when you are tensing a muscle and when you are relaxing it. By learning to distinguish the two, you can start to consciously control your muscular tension. Biofeedback practitioners can be found in your local yellow pages or the Alternative Medicine Yellow Pages.

References

The Alternative Medicine Yellow Pages
http://www.amazon.com or your local library

Personality

Unless you change your behavior, recurrence of your symptoms is inevitable... and your behavior is ultimately determined by your personality.

We Have Seen the Enemy... and it is us. Granted, everyone is different, but some traits are all too common among RSI sufferers. You are usually intense and hard-working, often stressed or obsessive, and almost always perfectionists. So it's not an easy task to lead you through a recovery process in which the fervor with which you attack your work must be regarded as the enemy. Your first step is acceptance... you are a compulsive worker. You must exorcise the compulsive part to save the worker part. Start now, your arms are too expensive.

Slow Down RSI is somewhat unpredictable, and in chronic cases, very confusing so it does not appeal to one's sense of logic. The first change you must make in your work habits is a reduction in the speed of work. The best you can do, with this in mind, is to make the changes gradually. Slowing down a little and not getting stressed out or working your fingers to the bone does not mean a lack of productivity. Learning to enjoy a few spare minutes of life besides work—and in conjunction with work—is not disloyalty to work. Taking micro-breaks and stretch breaks at work is not "goofing off." Remember, you are important. If your skill is valuable to an employer, it will be all the more dearly missed if you are completely disabled.

Think Through Problems If something gets you stressed out, figure out a solution that makes you comfortable. One very common problem observed in people recovering from RSI is the inner conflict because they can't satisfy everyone. Patients sometimes feel "boxed-in" to situations as they try to please someone else, but end up getting frustrated themselves. The key is to take decisive action and accept that you have done the best you can do, the right thing to do. Whatever decisions you've made, accept it and move on. Whatever you're concerned about, remind yourself that it's probably not as important to others as it is in your own mind.

Re-Evaluate Your Priorities   Your top priority is to stay healthy. If exercising is the only thing that is going to help you maintain your progress, make it a priority. This means making time during the day for exercises. You will never "find the time," you must *make the time*. If making the time means giving up something, decide on what you can give up and make the commitment. One excellent guidebook for blazing a new trail through life's choices is *Don't Sweat the Small Stuff* by Richard Carlson, Ph. D. It's full of simple, highly readable strategies that can help you un-stress your life.

Get a Therapist   A knowledgeable and caring therapist can support you, guide you, and help you understand the importance and logic of the various techniques used throughout the rehabilitation process. The rest is up to you.

References

Don't Sweat the Small Stuff
Richard Carlson, Ph. D., Hyperion, 1997

Warm Up Before Work

Establish a habit of warming up before working at the keyboard. Exactly what you settle on will be determined by what works for you. Here's a list of options:

- ❏   Wash your hands vigorously in warm water.
- ❏   Use a hand cream and rub it in until your hands are warm.
- ❏   Do finger stretches.
- ❏   Do our glide exercises on page 159.
- ❏   Take ten deep, abdominal breaths.
- ❏   Clench and open your hands 25 times.
- ❏   Do the rubber band exercises on page 149.
- ❏   Meditate.
- ❏   Do vision exercises, first focusing near you, then at a distance for a few seconds each.
- ❏   Massage your hands or forearms.
- ❏   Walk around or do some other mild aerobic activity to get your blood flowing.

Workstation Modification: Ergonomics

Each person is unique and your workstation should be equally individualized. In this section, we'll describe how to adjust your workstation precisely for the one person using it, you. The study of making the work environment conducive to human activities and the shape of the human body is called *ergonomics*. Ergonomic recommendations are often controversial, even though the basis for most of the ideas is usually "common-sensical." The problem is that too many recommendations seek to establish absolute, measurable guidelines, instead of staying focused on the underlying principles. With that warning in mind we present our over-riding goal for all of our ergonomic recommendations:

Our Golden Rule of Ergonomics

The objective is to work as much as possible in an unstressed position, with your upper body balanced, with the least muscle tension, and the lowest impact force. Any configuration or device that gets you closer to this goal is "good ergonomics" for you... irrespective of industry guidelines, rules-of-thumb, human factors averages, and so on. When we or anyone else cite specific dimensions or positions, it is just a starting point, based on what seems logical for a mythical, "average" person.

There Is No Perfect Setup   When you read anyone's ergonomic recommendations it's common to feel that one idea conflicts with another. For instance, we will say move close to the keyboard, and we will tell you not to bend your wrists. But you may find that the closer you move to the keyboard, the more you must bend your wrists! Yes, there are conflicts. One of the reasons we have this RSI problem is that there is no perfect position. Even if you get one of the fanciest ergonomic keyboards available, one that places the keys in a concave, curved alignment immediately at the tips of your fingers, not everyone's hand is the right size for the keyboard.

Moreover, the millions of repetitions mean that such a keyboard can arguably cause a more static position. More on that shortly.

Photos or Observation   If you've got a serious RSI problem, you really should have someone take some photos or at least watch you while you work. If you are getting rehabilitation, your therapist should perform a job site evaluation. It's very hard for you to honestly assess your own posture when you work, so someone else's perspective can be indispensable.

Your mission is to find the happy medium that lets you work with the least muscle tension. To do this, we'll consider each of the components of your workstation, one-by-one in the following sections.

> "The technique retraining is preventing me from re-injuring myself. I use 4-finger typing and major movements only. I also concentrate on my posture. I used to have horrible posture when typing. I also do not have my screen resolution set too small, so that I don't have to strain to see it. I would lean forward to see the smaller icons on the screen and ruin my posture."
>
> -- Patient A.

References

Challenging Conventional Ergonomics Wisdom
http://www.ur-net.com/office-ergo/conventi.htm
Credible, informed thinking from an ergonomist, debunking many commonly quoted ergonomic cliches.

The Overall Arrangement

Now that we've forewarned you that there is no single, ideal configuration for all people, we will present a generalized picture that sums up most of the current thinking on workstation arrangement. Keep in mind that the following picture does not encompass the "4th" dimension, "time." If you maintain even this idealized position too long, you'll have just as much trouble as if you ignore all of its lessons.

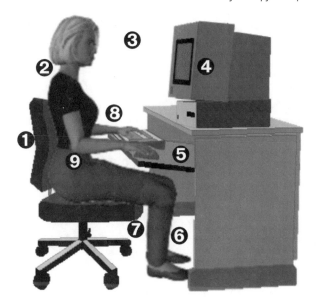

Proper Workstation Arrangement

This figure shows what you are trying to achieve in setting up your chair, desk, and computer. The rest of this chapter explains these items in detail. The numbers in the figure are explained below.

❶ Adjustable seat with good lumbar support.

❷ Posture comfortably balanced and upright.

❸ Monitor at the right reading distance for you.

❹ Monitor just below eye level, tilted up a little, free from glare.

❺ Keyboard and mouse on tray so you don't reach up to them; possibly tilted away from you slightly to avoid bending wrists up.

❻ Your feet reach the floor when your knees are at a 90-degree angle. Otherwise, use a footrest.

❼ Seat pan provides full support, no armrests.

❽ Forearms are horizontal so that the wrists are straight (left-to-right and up-down). Your wrist *do not rest on anything* when working.

❾ Elbows close by your side, so you don't have to support your arms. The bend should be slightly more open (closer to straight) than a 90-degree.

To accomplish the optimum setup for your circumstances, you'll have to start from the least changeable piece of equipment. In other words, if the keyboard simply must be at an awkward height, get a chair that lets you work with your arms horizontal and make your other adjustments from that position. Now let's look at each point in detail.

Chair

Your chair is no less important than the actual computer components of the workstation. Sometimes the chair is ignored because no one makes the connection between arm discomfort and posture. If your chair doesn't give you the support you need, or causes you to maintain an awkward posture, you'll develop the neck and shoulder fatigue that sets in motion the wheels of RSI.

Adjustability and Tilt The ideal chair is fully adjustable, including the seat pan, backrest, height, and arm rests. To encourage a balanced posture, the backrest should be tilted slightly forward and the seat pan tilted slightly down in front. Initially, this may give you a feeling that you are leaning forward slightly, but if your seat pan and backrest are the right size for you, you won't feel as if you're being thrown off your chair.

Height Chair height should be adjusted so that your feet can be flat on the floor with your hips and knees at roughly a 90-degree angle. Taller individuals should have a chair with a larger backrest and seat pan.

Armrests Armrests are optional. We recommend not having them, since they tend to cause pinch points while keyboarding, reducing blood flow. If you can discipline yourself to use arm rests only during rest times, there's nothing wrong with keeping them on. Make sure armrests are low enough that no elbow contact is made with them as you type.

Desk Surface and Keyboard Tray

Your desk and working space should be arranged with all the things you need within easy reach. You probably underestimate the frequency with which you perform routine activities. For example, consider the activity of answering the phone: if the phone is too far away, frequently reaching for it can aggravate your symptoms.

Height/ KeyboardTray The typical height of an office desk is conducive to writing but not to typing. For keyboarding and mouse use, a keyboard tray, attached to the bottom of the desk surface is recommended. It should be adjusted as close to the lap as possible, leaving enough space so that you can move your chair. There should be an inch or so of space between your legs and the tray. The keyboard tray should be tilted with the far end downward slightly, about 5-10 degrees. The goal of this so-called "negative tilt" is to is let your elbow form a comfortable angle, a little more than 90

The most widely used alternative keyboards are able to split in half and tilt to a greater or lesser degree. Here's a representative entry from the Kinesis company:

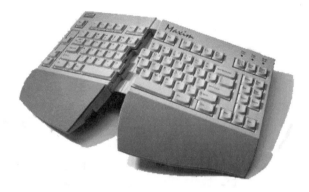

The Kinesis Maxim Keyboard

This alternative keyboard bends in the middle, so your wrists don't have to twist as much to meet the keys.

"I used the Comfort keyboard for a few months. It had three totally separate portions, one for the right and left parts of the main keyboard, and a third for the keypad. Each could be moved left or right wherever you wanted it and tilted at almost any angle or direction. There were times I thought it was curing me, and times I didn't. One definite problem with it, just like the conventional keyboards it replaces, is that the keys are in straight rows. So no matter what angle you place it at, some fingers have to stretch to reach the keys. For me it seemed like there was no perfect angle. Ultimately I had problems too serious for any keyboard to solve and I moved on to another workplace and back to a conventional keyboard."

--Patient E.

There are also keyboards that radically change the typing action, not just the position of the keys. One, called the Datahand, has a layout like a silhouette of your hands, with multi-purpose keys at each fingertip, to effect several letters or numbers. This means you hardly move your hands. Still others have the keys in curved, bowl-shaped rows to meet the fingers with less movement.

But is an alternative keyboard an improvement, even if it's not a full-fledged cure?

❑ *It would seem quite logical that* splitting the keyboard into halves, so the pieces are separated more would reduce ulnar deviation, allowing the wrist to be straighter.

❑ *It would seem quite logical that* tilting the keys up at the middle would reduce pronation, allowing the forearm to be less tense.

❑ *It would seem quite logical that* using a keyboard that reduces hand movement would reduce stress altogether.

You will only know by trying one, and perhaps trying it for at long time. Certainly, any design that gives you the same features you currently have, and adds adaptability and flexibility should be an improvement. If you can place the keys where your fingertips happen to fall in the neutral position, how could that hurt? Right?

The answer is *no one knows!* It's entirely possible that a keyboard that doesn't require your hands to move at all could do more harm than good. It depends on what you believe the big picture is—your big picture—and an accurate distinction between causes and results. If your problems have been caused by working in one position for ten years, you could argue that a single position keyboard is more problematic. Consider the following extrapolation of keyboard design "logic"... an argument by hyperbole. What if we design a keyboard with only one key. You press it once for "A," twice for "B," and so on. Ignore for a moment the inefficiency of typing letters toward the end of the alphabet, and consider the concept. You've eliminated awkward stretching, pronation, ulnar deviation, all that ugly stuff. But in two or three days, your forearm will swell up like a balloon. And if you're anything like the hundreds of Levi Strauss sewing machine operators who are routinely treated by our friend the Texas reflexologist, your triceps muscle will probably pinch off your ulnar nerve to the point of numbness in a matter of days. The point is that optimized keyboard design might reduce some stresses, but has three concerns you must be aware of:

❑ It conceivably can cause more repetition and static position, not less!

❑ It can initially make you feel great because you've shifted the stress to parts you haven't damaged yet. This might explain many of the glowing testimonials you read about the alternative keyboards.

❏ It can distract you from addressing the root cause: repetition and static position beyond your ability to cope.

We actually *do* believe the testimonials and we are generally *in favor of alternative keyboards*. But until better statistics are available, they are still in the realm of hopeful optimism. Bear in mind that better statistics will only arise when patients are followed for a period of at least one year. Given what we describe as a very murky situation, what can we say decisively about keyboard choices? Here's our bottom line:

❏ Any design that promotes the neutral position is better, as long as you have good blood flow and are in routine movement.

❏ A design that enables you to use less keystroke force—lower impact—is better.

❏ If you don't use the keypad much, consider getting a keyboard without one. This will let you move the mouse in closer, so you don't have to reach as far for it.

❏ The most wonderful keyboard in the world is not a solution, only a piece of the puzzle.

References

TI-FAQ, The Typing Injury FAQ
Exhaustive list of alternative keyboards, with reviews and photos.
http://www.tifaq.com/

Keyboard Alternatives & Vision Solutions
Supplier that offers trial periods on rental terms for a small fee, a nice option.
http://www.keyalt.com/
http://www.keyalt.com/kkeybrdp.htm

Key Layout

In the treatment section, we talked about typing with two fingers, or eliminating the use of the pinkies. If you're not ready to go to either of those extremes yet, you might investigate the possibility of altering the arrangement of keys on your keyboard.

The Qwerty Layout The normal layout, called the QWERTY layout, was actually designed to inconvenience you, so you would slow down. For those who haven't heard the story yet, the QWERTY layout was designed because touch typists of the past got so fast that they would constantly jam the old, mechanical keyboard mechanisms. As the story goes, one of the early typewriter makers concocted the least efficient layout to slow them down, and thus the QWERTY layout. Its organization makes common keystroke sequences especially awkward. But you can improve on this layout, if you're willing to learn a new layout.

The Dvorak Layout   The most well known alternative to the QWERTY layout is called the Dvorak layout, named for its creator. Microsoft Windows already has the Dvorak layout built in, and you can choose it by simply selecting Start Menu/Control Panel/Keyboard. The Dvorak layout reverses the QWERTY inefficiency by placing the most common keys on the "home" row, including all of the vowels on the fingers of the left hand, as shown here:

'	,	.	P	Y		F	G	C	R	L
A	O	E	U	I		D	H	T	N	S
;	Q	J	K	X		B	M	W	V	Z

While there is little doubt that the Dvorak layout fosters convenience, and therefore speed, it might not be the most comfortable or ergonomic. The main problem is that the small fingers are used as much as the large fingers, with the letter A on the left pinkie and S and L on the right.

The Bellis No-Pinkie Layout If you want to take the Dvorak technique one step further, you can remap the keys, meaning create your own arrangement. This is feasible by virtue of a keyboard generator program, such as the one shown here:

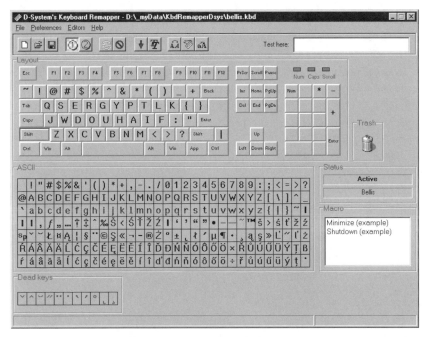

D-System's Keyboard Remapper

This class of utility program lets you create your own layout for the keyboard, so you can put the most common keys where your fingers are most at ease.

This program lets you create a new layout by simply dragging the letters from the grid at the bottom to the key you want them activated by, at the top. Based on various Web sites that analyze the frequency of letter usage in the language, we've come up with the following layout.

Q	S	E	R	G		Y	P	T	L	K
J	W	D	O	U		H	A	I	F	;
Z	X	C	V	B		N	M	,	.	/

The goal was to put the most used letters within easy reach of the large fingers, and change the notion of the "home row" so the fingers are not constantly bent as much. The gray keys in the chart represent the resting position of the fingers. With the middle and ring fingers on the top row, they don't bend as much.

With this layout, the greatest frequency of keystrokes occurs with very little use of the pinkies. After remapping the keys in this way, you can then move the actual plastic key caps to their new locations. With the computer off, pry them off and move them. (Note that some keyboards are not conducive to moving the keys because they have slightly different angles to the tops of the keys on each row—moving them will create a slightly bumpy layout.) Combined with the technique of removing the left Control key and emphasizing large movements for the numbers and combination keys, you can radically rebuild your entire typing habit.

References

Janko's Keyboard Generator
http://solair.eunet.yu/~janko/engdload.htm
Remaps the keys wherever you want. Free for non-commercial use. Windows 95 or 98.

D-System' Keyboard Remapper
http://www.kurt.hu/~marczi/keyboard.html
Remaps the keys wherever you want. $12 for personal use. For Windows 95, 98, or NT.

Typing Tutor
http://www. RSIProgram.com
A no-frills typing tutor game that will quickly teach you a new layout. In it, the letters drop from the top of the screen and you must press them before they hit the bottom.

The Mouse

Mice present an inevitable hazard because they require such fine and incessant positioning. Ironically (or is it?), it's the fact that they are so ideally suited to the task of pointing that makes them so damaging. That's because they get the job done with almost no motion whatsoever. For the user, however, this translates into static position and a constant pinching grasp. To combat this, we offer a combination of the same fundamentals that we recommend with keyboarding, and some specific ergonomic suggestions.

Use Your Arm Just as with the keyboard, try to use larger arm movements rather than twisting the wrist.

Straighten Your Wrist Make sure that the wrist is in line with the forearm and not bent up or down. If necessary, adjust your mouse tray or buy a new one. Particularly avoid an alignment that causes the pad of your hand to rest on the edge or corner of the work surface.

Stop Pinching Many people tend to hold the mouse with the tip of their thumb, clicking with the index finger. Instead, relax your thumb and let go of the "death grip." Try to simply rest your whole hand over the mouse and use both the index and middle fingers to click.

Mouse Trays Keyboard trays accommodate the mouse in one of two ways: some have one big flat surface for both the keyboard and mouse; others have a separate bracket attachment tray for the mouse. Ideally, the mouse should be at the same level as the keyboard, suggesting that one flat surface is preferred. With this configuration, you can put the whole tray at a slight negative angle (downward at the far edge) for the mouse as well, enabling you to keep your wrist straight. This single surface configuration also makes it easier to change the mouse from side to side to use with either hand, distributing the load between them. However, if you become accustomed to working with your keyboard at a significant negative angle, the mouse becomes a nuisance, sliding off all the time. Your only recourse if you do choose this type of keyboard tray is to arrange a platform for the mouse, propped up at the back with something like a small towel. A low-tech way to make the platform is to use ½" thick foam core board, available from a framing shop or art supply store, and tape it in position with strong tape.

Move the Mouse In If you don't need the numeric keypad of your keyboard, install a brand of keyboard that does not have a keypad in it. Then you can bring the mouse closer to you, thereby relieving some of the stress on the arm that uses the mouse. If you have a keyboard tray with a separate mouse platform, you may be able to rotate the mouse platform in over the top of the numeric keypad.

Connect Two Mice at Once With a device called a Y-Mouse™ Dual Mouse Adapter, you can have two different types of mice—as long as they can work with the same software driver—connected at the same time. You might use a regular mouse for graphics and use the trackball, which requires less pinching, for all other tasks. Alternating between them reduces the monotonous position. It is about $45 because it includes some electronics.

> "I've moved the mouse to the left (even though I'm right-handed) because, with no number pad on the left, it's closer on that side. This way, I don't have to reach as far and I create less tension in my shoulder and chest."
>
> -- Patient F.

Swap Sides Consider switching the mouse from side to side every few weeks.

> *We offer this recommendation with a healthy dose of caution: use this technique only after you've learned to manage your body's response to RSI. Simply switching hands to try to escape from symptoms that you haven't gained any control over will only lead to more damage.*

It's not easy getting started with the mouse on the "wrong" side, but with practice, you'll be just as efficient. Remember, don't push either side to the point of fatigue. The idea is to distribute the workload, not to cause injury to both sides!

Which Mouse is the Best? No mouse is a "good" mouse—they all cause overuse of different groups of muscles. The only mouse that won't hurt you is one that you don't use to do repetitive tasks! People have varying success with alternate mouse styles such as trackballs, pens, and touchpads, and you should certainly investigate them if you have serious problems using a mouse. Even some conventional mice simply have a better shape that reduces the pinching action. Trackballs can also reduce the pinching action, but will initially be awkward for high-power word processing or programming. Pressure sensitive touch pads or graphics tablets are an option for some users. These are built into many laptop computers, but can be purchased separately. With these devices, you use either your fingertip or a pen on a surface that reads your position.

"I now use an ergonomic chair that has an adjustable back and seat pan tilt, and no arms. I also use an adjustable height table, an adjustable height keyboard tray, a split keyboard, a Cirque Glidepoint instead of a mouse, a telephone headset, a document holder, a book stand, and a voice recognition system "Dragon Naturally Speaking." My keyboard is called Options by IBM, (previously the Lexmark Select Ease). This keyboard splits completely in half which allows me to place the Glidepoint in between the two sections. This setup has helped me enormously."

-- Patient D.

"The Cirque Glidepoint is fabulous."

-- Patient C.

Evaluating Mice   Your first criteria in evaluating a new mouse will probably be whether you can use it productively, irrespective of any comfort considerations. For instance, you may find a trackball unsuited to graphics work. Only after you find a mouse that works will you try to judge whether it is less stressful. This is a difficult judgment to make since the mere act of changing to a different mouse, aside from of the relative long term merits of the two styles, might cause more discomfort as you concentrate on the new techniques. If so, you may not give it a fair chance. Conversely, it's possible that the new one will feel better initially because it uses different muscles. Then, as your capacity is exceeded on these muscles, your symptoms recur.

So, unless you have a compelling reason to change the type of mouse, get a high quality, conventional mouse, sized comfortably for your hand... make sure it is properly situated... and learn to use it as we've described.

Reference

Cirque Cruise Cat and Glidepoint Touchpads
http://www.cirque.com

Dual Mouse Y-Adapter
PI Engineering, Inc., available from http://www.cdw.com

The Telephone

Cradling the telephone between the shoulder and neck is one of the worst things you can do to your neck. Although software developers probably don't *get* RSI from the phone, habitual phone misuse can definitely be an aggravating factor once you have a serious RSI problem. For tech-support and customer service personnel, however, cradling a phone all day can be a primary cause of RSI. Remember that many people get their first symptoms in the neck and shoulder.

Speakerphone or Headset   When you talk on the phone, try using the speaker-phone whenever possible. If you use the phone constantly, get a headset. Wireless ones are now available. Attachments to a telephone receiver that let you sit the phone on your shoulder *do not help*. They often do not fit properly, requiring you to lift your shoulder to hold the receiver in place.

Use Phone Time Proactively   Telephone time is good to use as a reminder for posture correction and performance of some simple stretches, even standing up and pacing around in your office space.

Get Your Money's Worth

Don't expect to be able to decide if you like any new workstation equipment in just a few days of use. Plan to try things out for about a month. If you find that it is not comfortable, try another one. We've become accustomed to large retailers offering liberal money-back exchange policies for their products, but ergonomic equipment suppliers have not quite gotten to that point yet. If you shop around, however, you can find suppliers that will give you enough options that you can try out ergonomic equipment without bearing all of the risk. Try to find a supplier that has a liberal return policy or a rental period. As an RSI patient, it's important to make full use of such policies. Remember, the manufacturers and retailers of all those awkward products that helped to get you into trouble in the first place never gave a second thought to your problems. Even if you don't feel they "owe you" anything, it's in the supplier's best interest to get you to try out their products. Demanding that they—instead of you—carry the risk is a simple matter of balancing the scales by negotiating for your fair share. The financial loss of an occasional item returned to them is not an undue hardship if you return a product in saleable condition. Search the web for ergonomic suppliers and compare their purchase terms.

Part 5: Organized Prevention

The Challenge of the Road Less Traveled

Prevention is both the most important of all RSI topics and the most challenging. To appreciate its importance, you need only talk to RSI sufferers and hear the unanimous pleas for a second chance… to be able to set the clock back and start all over again. Every one of them would have you believe that they would be more diligent in taking breaks, getting more diverse activity, and working with better attention to posture and form. But try to sell these concepts to young, healthy workers who are at a point in life where they're obsessed with the passion for accomplishment and equally convinced that they're invincible, and you'll see what a hard sell it is. Because RSI has no single event to attach to it… because it affords no concrete, easily recognized measurement, and because of the sorry state of information about it, RSI makes a poor basis for the prevention sales pitch.

Throughout this book, you've read about the many problems of RSI politics: the erroneous stigma of RSI sufferers as malingerers, the misunderstanding by conventional medical practitioners, the misconceptions of the general public, and to this day, the relative uncertainty of all RSI information—ours included. To this sad mix, you must add the primary motivation that drives the policy of most employers. No, it's not money. It's fear. They're afraid that dealing with RSI head-on will open the floodgates of medical claims, and the "con artists" and disgruntled workers will come pouring through. Finally, even the insurance companies—those who you would think have the most to gain by being proactive—appear to be taking the ostrich stance on things, sticking their heads in the sand. They're satisfied to ride the status quo because they don't actually gamble on odds; they simply calculate what's called recent "experience" in actuarial tables and pass all expenses on to the customer, ultimately us.

With this difficult landscape spread out in front of us, we nonetheless strongly encourage you and your organization to develop and promote an RSI prevention program. With computers becoming a way of life, and doing so at preschool ages, preventive programs are desperately important. If you, perhaps an RSI sufferer, want your company to start a prevention program, it may take extensive education of "the powers that be." They have to be convinced that it is a serious health problem, and that starting such a program makes sense financially.

Whether you are an individual in a small setting, or a corporate policy maker, the stakes are human as well as monetary. Should RSI prevention be pursued because it makes long-term monetary sense for your company, or should you do it because it's important to prevent human suffering? Only you can decide. In a corporate setting, what probably matters most is which line of reasoning has the most appeal to the person who will ultimately sponsor your program. From our point of view, however, any program that is motivated *solely* by "cost-justification," or a so-called "business case" will eventually run out of steam and fail because the commitment is not as persistent as the opposition. The opposition is RSI, and it is a tough, long-term problem. It has endless patience, it is pervasive, and it has all the factors in its favor: increasing division of labor, intense competition, shortening work cycles and deadlines, and so on.

With so formidable an opponent, superficial motives—despite the presumed appeal of financial payback—probably won't be sufficient. Instead, someone in a key decision making role must truly care about co-workers as people and believe that investing in people is simply the right thing to do. We believe that only an attitude of genuine caring and responsibility will provide a long-lasting foundation for a successful RSI prevention program. Your challenge is to find the person who cares. A preventive program cannot be half-hearted.

So what is the formula for a successful program at a high-risk company? In designing an effective prevention program, the following aspects must be addressed:

- ❏ Designing a program that fosters not just words but action
- ❏ Educating those at risk and their superiors
- ❏ Improving workstation ergonomics
- ❏ Reducing body vulnerability and improving flexibility, strength, endurance, and general fitness
- ❏ Improving work habits and the corporate culture: encouraging early intervention

About Those Floodgates When you begin your program, yes, the floodgates will appear to burst open with RSI patients. Don't lose your resolve—it's a normal reaction. There are many individuals who genuinely have minor aches and pains, and your program should draw them out and identify their situation as just that... minor. Along with those "false positives," (to use the doctors' term) you will invariably find a few individuals who are on their way to developing a serious RSI problem. By encouraging them to deal with the problem early, you may very well save them from years of misery. In doing so, you will distinguish your organization as one where people really count, and make it one that people genuinely want to be a part of. In today's employment market, we believe such a practice is just good business.

Where to Put Your Emphasis The following sections will look at each of the above topics in detail. As you'll see, however, we'll recommend that you place the greatest emphasis on early intervention, getting people to report symptoms and address them before they become serious. That's because the people whom you're most likely to have any impact on are those who've noticed some symptoms. The other aspects of the program are certainly important, but until people become somewhat vulnerable, education and good advice only go so far. The most likely effect of information is awareness, not substantial changes in behavior. Early intervention, on the other hand, has a highly leveraged effect. By intercepting symptoms before one's nervous system is involved or extensive muscular inflammation occurs, you can keep people away from the danger zone of chronic RSI and its protracted recovery periods.

An RSI Prevention Program

Anyone can point you to decent information on RSI. Putting that information into "actionable" tasks is the hard part. Here are our ideas on how to cross the bridge from passive knowledge to active prevention.

Map Out A Plan

Step 1: Get Top Management Support   If a program does not have the genuine support of the highest level of your operating unit, don't even consider proceeding. Sadly, it usually takes a serious RSI loss (an injured employee) to open the channels of communication with top management, but so be it. Talk to the president or vice president as the case may be, and ask him or her to let you deal with the problem head-on instead of waiting for the next surprise.

Step 2: Find a Motivated Owner of the Program   Once you've got management support, someone has to "own" the RSI problem, from a prevention point of view. The owner makes all of the activities of the program occur. You might start your hunt in the HR department, or maybe it's you.

Step 3: Choose a Workstation Advisor   This is someone who will advise workers on improving the ergonomics of their workstation and make them aware of the resources available, including items such as keyboard trays, chairs and so on. More details are described in the upcoming topic on *Workstation Ergonomics*.

Step 4: Choose Healthcare Professionals   Decide who your "primary diagnostician" will be for RSI patients. This could be anyone in the healthcare chain of command who has been successful at evaluating RSI situations: a nurse, physical therapist, doctor, orthopedic surgeon, alternative therapist, or perhaps an ergonomist.

If your primary diagnostician is not a physician, you will also need a physician as part of the system. This physician need not be on site, but certainly needs to understand RSI and the philosophy of the prevention program. Because RSI doesn't mesh neatly into the cogs of today's healthcare machinery, you must carefully select a doctor who demonstrates a strong commitment to solving RSI problems.

More and more, it is the physical therapists who are taking the lead in the battle against RSI, so we believe a physical therapist with extensive RSI experience is a key ingredient in any program. The PT can render advice regarding exercises and workstation modifications, and can provide hands-on treatment as necessary.

Step 5: Conduct a Survey Send out surveys to determine the current state of affairs in your company. We believe people are somewhat overwhelmed with surveys, so keep it short and to the point. Here's a complete sample survey:

Repetitive Strain Injury Survey

The following questions are being asked of all employees in anticipation of setting up a prevention program for Repetitive Strain Injuries (which many people know of by its most popularized subtype, carpal tunnel syndrome).

Questions? Contact _____, RSI Prevention Coordinator

❑ Yes   ❑ No   Do your hands, arms, shoulders, or neck hurt when you type?

❑ Yes   ❑ No   Do you feel tingling, numbness, or cold fingers?

❑ Yes   ❑ No   Do you find yourself stretching or massaging after a few hours of keyboard work?

❑ Yes   ❑ No   Have you switched hands for certain computer tasks?

❑ Yes   ❑ No   Have you been woken by hand numbness when sleeping?

❑ Yes   ❑ No   Have you been typing more than 7 years?

❑ Yes   ❑ No   Is your workstation as comfortable as you would like?

❑ Yes   ❑ No   Would you like more information or assistance with regard to ergonomics or typing injuries?

Name _____

Step 6: Create Literature Decide what information you want to focus on and prepare handouts to use during your training sessions. You might want to have information on RSI basics, stretches, exercises, and workstation ergonomics, at the minimum. We recommend that you *not* resort to simply handing out literature in a mass mailing. This might be perceived as a Band Aid approach that could trivialize the problem and undermine an otherwise sincere attempt to deal with it. Instead hand out the literature to those who attend your training sessions. You can, however, include some of the basics in your employee orientation literature. Don't include diagnostic or therapeutic information in orientation literature—that's too detailed for a general audience.

Step 7: Schedule and Conduct Training Set up ergonomic training sessions for new and existing employees. For existing employees, it might be by department (regardless of symptom occurrence), or grouped by level of symptoms reported on the survey. Training sessions will be most effective if performed by an employee of the company, from the safety or ergonomic department if the company is large enough, along with the primary diagnostician in your system. Distribute the handouts you've created. More details are described in the next section, *Education*.

Step 8: Provide Individual Consultation Employees with distinct RSI symptoms should be given one-on-one sessions with your "primary diagnostician" to evaluate their condition. If there are many employees with symptoms, give priority to those with constant or severe symptoms, and adjust your plan after getting some initial feedback from the diagnostician. Refer individuals with significant pain or any nerve symptoms to appropriate medical professionals. Every effort must be made to prevent employees with serious symptoms from returning to a full workload until they are treated, because advanced problems are very slow to reverse.

The following sections will explain the key elements of the program in more detail.

Education

Include an RSI segment in your orientation training of newly hired employees. For existing staff, schedule sessions as needed to present the same information until everyone has gotten the message.

Orientation Training Although the subject could easily take up to three hours, you can't expect a healthy ("non-symptomatic") audience to have much patience for RSI lecturing. For orientation training, try to cover just the basics in 15-20 minutes, and offer optional resources for those who want more information. For existing employees, a half-hour to an hour is reasonable, and could certainly be adjusted if you've grouped the audience according to how much at risk they are, or if they have symptoms already. The goal of this level of training is awareness, not correction. Cover the following topics in your basic RSI training:

❑ **Introduction** Explain the purpose and components of the RSI Prevention Program:

   ❑ The purpose of the program is to prevent injury from an increasingly predictable problem.

   ❑ The program will consist of education, ergonomic recommendations and equipment, early intervention, actively involved RSI experts, the work culture, and employee participation.

❑ **Overview of RSI** Provide an Overview of RSI, explaining how it occurs, what the symptoms are, and how it can be controlled:

   ❑ Repetitive Strain Injury is muscle and/or nerve problems caused by incessant work in a single posture, with highly repetitive actions, such as typing. It wasn't as much of a problem with typewriters because typewriters had steeply stepped rows of keys, requiring you to hold your hands up, and there was a lot more variety of motion using a typewriter. Rarely could someone work dawn-'til-dusk typing, let alone with their hands in one position, but we do now.

   ❑ Symptoms include pain, burning, numbness, tingling in the fingers or arms; a constant need to stretch or massage one's arms; or fatigue when working. Carpal Tunnel Syndrome is the name for one type of RSI that involves swelling in the wrist. Computer users get RSI problems at any point from their back and neck down to their fingertips. *Explain that most RSI cases are not serious... we are instituting a program because serious cases are avoidable.*

   ❑ RSI is controlled by a wide range of techniques depending on the specific symptoms and extent of damage. For initial, minor symptoms, physical improvements to the workstation, called ergonomics, suffice. For more serious cases, work habits must be changed substantially, often including posture and breaks. For chronic cases, massage and other physical therapies are also used.

❑ **Report Early** Explain that the company is committed first-and-foremost to reducing the likelihood of chronic RSI and that the single most important step in accomplishing that is early intervention. This means that employees who are experiencing any RSI-related symptoms should report them to the human resources department or nurse immediately. Highlight this point prominently so people remember it:

Our Top Priority

The top priority of our program is
to recognize and deal with RSI symptoms as early as possible,
so that minor problems do not develop into serious ones.

❑ **We Are Proactive** Explain that reporting work-related health problems is not viewed negatively by the company, and that it is to the employee's advantage to report the problem at work because they will get help directly from an RSI expert. If, in trying to avoid having a "recordable" work injury they seek help on their own, they may lose crucial time visiting doctors who are not well-versed on RSI. Some may not even recommend any treatment or remediation. The earlier you catch RSI, the easier it is to treat, so losing time can be a crucial mistake.

❑ **The Initial Hysteria** Explain that it's normal to have an initial wave of reported problems at the beginning of the program, but it's not because RSI is psychologically contagious. It's because many of us work through minor pains that don't become serious. Raising awareness of RSI will initially make us notice and report more of these aches and pains.

❑ **Relate Prevention in Real Terms** To instill the importance of prevention, provide "real world" examples of how RSI has affected the day-to-day lives of some co-workers. It's human nature to believe that we're invincible and that "it won't happen to me," so the material discussed during these meetings is not always taken seriously. The success of the RSI program depends upon the employees believing that this is indeed a problem, and their willingness to work together to prevent it.

Targeted RSI Training   Periodically present more detailed RSI sessions specifically for individuals who have reported symptoms in response to your survey. The general employee population can also be invited on a purely voluntary basis. These sessions can be at lunchtime if necessary, for a half-hour to an hour. Include the following topics, above and beyond those in the orientation training:

- ❏   Setting up an ergonomically comfortable workstation.
- ❏   Posture and neutral position.
- ❏   The need for breaks and tools for reminding you to take them.
- ❏   Stretching and strengthening exercises.
- ❏   Detecting localized syndromes (e.g., tendinitis), spasms, and trigger points.
- ❏   Recognizing susceptibility factors for serious RSI: non-stop work intensity, perfectionism, and obsession.
- ❏   Distinguishing telltale signs of chronic RSI: loss of sleep, numbness, etc.
- ❏   Other therapy options: massage, yoga, biofeedback, etc.

Supervisory Training   Include in your existing supervisory training a ten-minute segment on RSI. Explain the following RSI points:

- ❏   Emphasize that managers need to be on the lookout for individuals who are high-risk. The risk factors are not in any way conclusive, but they are fairly well confirmed by RSI sufferers. In other words, some people have all of these factors but never get RSI. RSI sufferers on the other hand almost always have some of these factors: incessant keyboarding; perfectionism; highly bent wrists; slouching posture; many years at the computer; neck pushed forward as if straining to see the monitor; no exercise; high stress.
- ❏   Work expectations, deadlines, and attitude must be managed so that constant time at the keyboard is not perceived as the only priority at the workplace.
- ❏   Supervisors share the responsibility for improving the ergonomics of employees' workstations.

Workstation Ergonomics and Supplies

Provide an "Expert" There are two parts to promoting better workstation ergonomics: equipment and the expertise to implement it. If you have a large organization, you'll probably already have someone under whose job responsibilities ergonomics might naturally fall. If not, either train a key employee who wants to learn some basic ergonomics, or provide access to someone who is already informed on the issues.

The objective here is not to get too complicated, but instead to stick to the basics: the goal is to help workers achieve a workstation that is highly adaptable to their proportions, and work in the neutral position. This simply means a balanced posture, arms not outstretched very far, and comfortably straight wrists. Trying to do much more than that gets into the realm of professional ergonomics and is not necessarily better, since many ergonomic concepts are the subject of much debate.

Establish a Purchasing Procedure Arrange terms with two or three ergonomic suppliers with the stipulation that equipment can be returned within a certain timeframe. Wherever possible, establish a small number of standard, preferred item styles. For instance, there might be one or two preferred styles of alternative keyboard. For keyboard trays, because they will be fastened to desks, it can be advantageous to settle on a single style, so that all workstations are roughly interchangeable. The goal is to have easy access to equipment and arrive at a uniformly adaptable workstation configuration for all employees in the company. A priority list may have to be established so that the most symptomatic individuals get the equipment first.

Maintain a Small Inventory If you have more than 100 employees, establish a small inventory of general ergonomic equipment, including at the minimum:

- Keyboard trays

- Foot rests

- Monitor stands

Reminder Software Keep copies of reminder software on your network, and publicize it in your RSI literature. Refer to *Tools, Supplies, Software* on page 103 for sources.

Reduce Body Vulnerability

Body vulnerability is "owned" by the employee alone, and no one can do the work for them. It refers to overall physical fitness (strength, endurance, and flexibility), diet, sleep, and mental resilience. Although the employer can't do the work for the employees, plenty can be done to help. Here are some suggestions:

❑   Organize extracurricular activities, or at least provide the means for employees to organize them. For instance, put up a bulletin board just for activities. Make an e-mail distribution list for activities. Notice we're not limiting the concept to strictly sports. Any activities will help.

❑   Include flexibility, strength, and endurance exercises in the literature you hand out in your RSI training sessions.

❑   Larger sites can provide onsite workout facilities. Aerobics, yoga, and weight control sessions may be beneficial.

❑   Institute a fitness reimbursement plan or discount for health club membership.

Foster Good Work Habits and Behavior

"Good work habits and behavior" means not keyboarding incessantly... having some variety to your tasks... and not feeling oppressed by one's work. Although you could argue that these are all behaviors solely under the control of the employee, they are substantially the result of the work culture fostered by the company. Even for employees that are self-motivated workaholics, the employer might be facilitating the obsessive keyboarding habit to a certain extent. And some work environments unintentionally foster a never-ending cycle of crushing deadlines or a sense of urgency to the work that is simply unjustified by realities.

Instituting change at this level, the organizational culture, is one of the toughest challenges and most difficult areas for concrete recommendations. There is no bullet list of easy-to-do techniques. Managers are understandably consumed with meeting deadlines and achieving productivity goals. Employees' habits are very resistant to change and personality is very ingrained, so employees who are prone to obsessive keyboarding won't change much by simply being told what's good for them.

This type of change, if it's necessary can only come from the chain of command, meaning at or near the top... at least from the top of a business unit. If your organization has a serious RSI problem and it is a high-stress, constant deadline workplace, the problem might not have started at the top, but the solution must. Top management must send a new message—and the actions to go with it—down through the ranks. The message must convey that more wholesome decision making will be valued for its long-term benefits. Managers must become aware of trends that put workers at a high-risk for RSI and strive to minimize the dangers.

RSI Prevention for Students

Our focus throughout this book has been on hard-core computer users, especially those with chronic RSI or the potential for it, so school students have not been mentioned much. However, viewing the problem "from 40-thousand feet," the potential for chronic RSI is more severe in our schools than anywhere else. We're not going to try to fully cover the topic of prevention for students, but we do want to map out our concepts as they apply to young people. With that goal, we offer the following synopsis of our theory as a checklist for school faculty members, parents, and college students. We've made every effort to keep our suggestions realistic and down-to-earth, so you have a real chance to put them into action.

Overall Behavior

The goal is to keep your arms in motion, and to give your body the chance to repair the normal wear-and-tear of work. Computer use, sustained for long periods of time, is surprisingly hard work, and it is the unnatural, unmoving posture that causes the damage.

- ❏ Don't type for hours at a time.

- ❏ Ideally, students under 12 shouldn't use the computer for more than one hour per day.

- ❏ Get well-rounded physical activity and regular exercise.

- ❏ If you use the computer more than one hour per day, you must take breaks. Take a 2-5 minute break every 15-30 minutes of work.

- ❏ Don't just sit there! Walk around to think, use a whiteboard or blackboard, write notes or diagrams on cards.

Positioning Techniques

<u>The goal</u> is to work in low-stress, "neutral" positions. Neutral positions are those in which the joints are most relaxed and the posture is balanced. By balancing the posture, you work with as little muscle tension as possible.

- ❑ If you're typing for more than a few minutes, make sure you sit up straight. Many RSI problems result from years of sitting with the shoulders curled forward, usually because of fatigue.

- ❑ Keep your wrists straight.

- ❑ Don't rest your wrists on a wrist pad or the edge of a desk. When typing, your hands should be suspended.

- ❑ Keep your elbows close by your side. Don't reach out. Reaching creates muscle tension.

- ❑ The more you type, the more you must learn to reach the keys by moving your whole arm, not just contorting your hand and fingers.

- ❑ Use a light touch while typing.

- ❑ Don't pinch the mouse forcefully. When you can, use a touchpad.

- ❑ Using a laptop computer on top of a desk is one of the worst possible arrangements because the wrists are usually bent and pinched. If you must do so, don't type for hours at a time.

- ❑ For lengthy prose like term papers, use voice recognition software.

- ❑ When you're thinking, not typing, rest your hands in your lap.

Workstation

<u>The goal</u> is to make your workstation match your neutral, unstressed position. You shouldn't have to adapt to your workstation.

- ❑ Don't put computer keyboards on desks that are intended for writing. Use a keyboard tray to lower the keyboard so your arms are at a relaxed height and your shoulders are not hunched up.

- ❑ Position your monitor so you don't have to lean forward to see it.

- ❑ Use a properly sized chair, so your feet reach the floor and your back is against the chair.

- ❑ Your chair should not have armrests. If it does, don't rest your arms on them when typing.

- ❑ Place the mouse as close to you as possible, so you don't reach out.

The Last Word

Perhaps by now you've realized that I, Jack Bellis, am the pseudonymous "Patient E." We've hardly gone out of our way to disguise that fact. I'm the one that required 21 sessions of therapy to break down the knots on my ulnar nerve. My current status is what I would call "manageable." That is, I can control my symptoms while I work. I have only one persistent symptom that I haven't completely kicked, a little pinching sensation when I type for long sessions. I do warm-ups, stretches, and take breaks to work without causing more damage. My tolerance for keyboarding is steadily, but slowly increasing—I've had periods of as long as three weeks where I've worked completely symptom-free. I am vulnerable, but not a victim.

In retrospect I believe that having worked through pain for several months (years ago), ignorant of the damage I was doing, was my big mistake. If you take away from this book only one thing, just as we have said with our prevention program, it's the thought that you should address RSI symptoms early.

The only reason I'm not a victim is that a dedicated therapist, Suparna Damany, was willing to fight against much resistance to bring her knowledge and concern to our company. She had seen many people suffer excessively with RSI, and two of my co-workers were among them. She helped one of them, our Patient A., recover from repeated, painful mistreatment at the hands of less-informed practitioners, and made her well again. The other employee, a manager whom Suparna had also helped, waged a personal war to help Suparna establish a presence at our company. This is when I came under her treatment. I suspect that if Suparna and the manager had not shown the guts that they did, the two small fingers on my left hand would be non-functional right now. In an all-too-predictable turn of events, a business change occurred and Suparna's on-site physical therapy was quietly discontinued. Someone was afraid.

I stopped by a co-worker's cubicle recently to show him how to edit some icons, and saw that he had switched his mouse to the other hand... for the second time in a few months. After the first episode, he returned the mouse to the original hand and was optimistic that he had solved what would prove to be a minor problem. At the time of the first episode, I avoided "interfering"—I just told him a little of the concept of working in the most neutral position. But it makes me painfully aware of the other thing I hope you will take away from this book: a little courage to deal head-on with this very mischievous RSI phenomenon. Don't play doctor, but don't stick your head in the sand either. People out there need help and you might be the only one they encounter with enough information to steer them in the right direction.

I think I'll go have a talk with my friend editing those icons.

Index

Warm Up and Break Reminder

Copy this page as much as you want and post near workstations.

Warm up: wash your hands in warm water, massage your arms, rub in hand cream.

Exhale Relax

www.RSIProgram.com

RSI Prevention and Treatment at a Glance

Copy this page as much as you want and post near workstations.

All Typists and First-Degree RSI Patients, Those with Erratic Aches

Keep your wrists straight.

Don't rest your wrists on a wrist pad.

Use a properly sized chair with lumbar support.

Keep your elbows close by your side. Don't reach out.

Take a 2-5 minute break every 15-30 minutes of work.

Use a keyboard tray so your arms are at a relaxed height.

Reach the keys by moving your whole arm, not just your hand.

Balance your shoulders and head above your torso. Don't slouch forward.

Second-Degree RSI Patients, Those with Predictable Aches and Pains

Warm up.

Stretch frequently.

Perform "glide" exercises.

Exercise your whole body.

Avoid combination keystrokes.

Strengthen your entire upper extremity.

Breathe by pushing your stomach in and out.

Reduce your typing until you control your symptoms.

See a healthcare professional.

Get more sleep.

Third-Degree RSI Patients, Those with Numbness or Constant Pain

Stop typing until you control your symptoms.

Get professional massage to eliminate muscle spasms or trigger points.

Temporarily type with one or three fingers on each hand.

Become less obsessive about keyboard work.

Get started with voice recognition software.

Try yoga or biofeedback.

www.RSIProgram.com